AF439914

Histopathology of Chronic Constipation

William A. Meier-Ruge, Basel
Elisabeth Bruder, Basel

105 figures, 93 in color, 6 tables, 2012

KARGER

Basel · Freiburg · Paris · London · New York · New Delhi · Bangkok ·
Beijing · Tokyo · Kuala Lumpur · Singapore · Sydney

Prof. William A. Meier-Ruge
Institut für Pathologie der Universität Basel
Schönbeinstrasse 40
CH–4031 Basel (Switzerland)
E-Mail meier-ruge@bluewin.ch

PD Dr. Elisabeth Bruder
Institut für Pathologie der Universität Basel
Schönbeinstrasse 40
CH–4031 Basel (Switzerland)
E-Mail elisabeth.bruder@unibas.ch

Second revised edition of Meier-Ruge WA, Bruder E: Pathology of Chronic Constipation in Pediatric and Adult Coloproctology. Basel, Karger, 2005.

For this book the authors thank for the generous financial support of the Freiwillige Akademische Gesellschaft Basel.

Library of Congress Cataloging-in-Publication Data

Meier-Ruge, W. (William)
 Histopathology of chronic constipation / William A. Meier-Ruge, Elisabeth
Bruder. -- 2nd rev. ed.
    p. ; cm.
 Rev. ed. of: Pathology of chronic constipation in pediatric and adult
coloproctology / William A. Meier-Ruge, Elizabeth Bruder. 2005.
 Includes bibliographical references and index.
 ISBN 978-3-318-02174-5 (hard cover : alk. paper) -- ISBN 978-3-318-02175-2
(electronic)
 I. Bruder, Elisabeth. II. Meier-Ruge, W. (William). Pathology of chronic
constipation in pediatric and adult coloproctology. III. Title.
 [DNLM: 1. Chronic Disease. 2. Constipation--pathology. 3. Colonic
Diseases--diagnosis. 4. Diagnosis, Differential. WI 409]

 616.3'4280472--dc23
          2012023033

S. Karger
Medical and Scientific Publishers
Basel · Freiburg · Paris · London · New York ·
New Delhi · Bangkok · Beijing · Tokyo ·
Kuala Lumpur · Singapore · Sydney

Disclaimer
The statements, opinions and data contained in this publication are solely those of the individual authors and contributors and not of the publisher and the editor(s). The appearance of advertisements in the journal is not a warranty, endorsement, or approval of the products or services advertised or of their effectiveness, quality or safety. The publisher and the editor(s) disclaim responsibility for any injury to persons or property resulting from any ideas, methods, instructions or products referred to in the content or advertisements.

Drug Dosage
The authors and the publisher have exerted every effort to ensure that drug selection and dosage set forth in this text are in accord with current recommendations and practice at the time of publication. However, in view of ongoing research, changes in government regulations, and the constant flow of information relating to drug therapy and drug reactions, the reader is urged to check the package insert for each drug for any change in indications and dosage and for added warnings and precautions. This is particularly important when the recommended agent is a new and/or infrequently employed drug.

All rights reserved.
No part of this publication may be translated into other languages, reproduced or utilized in any form or by any means, electronic or mechanical, including photocopying, recording, microcopying, or by any information storage and retrieval system, without permission in writing from the publisher or, in the case of photocopying, direct payment of a specified fee to the Copyright Clearance Center (see 'General Information').

© Copyright 2012 by S. Karger AG,
P.O. Box, CH–4009 Basel (Switzerland)
Printed in Germany
on acid-free and non-aging paper (ISO 9706) by
Bosch-Druck GmbH, Ergolding
ISBN 978–3–318–02174–5
e-ISBN 978–3–318–02175–2

KARGER

Fax +41 61 306 12 34
E-Mail karger@karger.ch
www.karger.com

Contents

Contents

Foreword

In 2005, the *Journal of Pathobiology* (vol. 72) published a review about the pathohistology of motility disorders of the gut. This publication about the morphology of chronic constipation had a remarkable echo. Now, 7 years later, it seemed to be the time to write an update so as to incorporate the new data which has become available since that review. This book represents more than 40 years of experience in rectocolic biopsy diagnostics of gut motility disorders. Pathologists will find much diagnostic information in the field of chronic constipation, often considered as a functional disease without a morphological substrate.

It became obvious that not only an aganglionosis (Hirschsprung's disease), but also a lack or atrophy of the tendinous collagen net in circular and longitudinal muscles may cause an aperistaltic syndrome.

Enzyme histochemistry has proven to be the pathophysiological technique of choice in the pathology of chronic constipation. This method provides insights into gastrointestinal motility disorders by the cholinergic nervous system and the dehydrogenase activity of nerve cells in the submucous and myenteric plexus. The dehydrogenases of the citric circle selectively stain nerve cells in the intestinal wall. Nitroxide synthase helps the pathologist in immediate sections for microscopic examination under surgery to reliably inform the pediatric surgeon whether the planned resection margin is aganglionic, hypoganglionic, or normal innervated.

Enzyme histochemistry overcomes the often frustrating results of classical histological stainings in formalin-fixed biopsies. Besides classical Hirschsprung's disease, it is also possible to differentiate in mucosal biopsies ultrashort Hirschsprung's disease, immaturity of the enteric nervous system, and neuronal dysplasia.

A laboratory guide provides instructions on how to prepare colorectal biopsies or surgical specimens, and how to transport them to the histopathological laboratory over long distances. The most important enzyme histochemical reactions in the diagnosis of gastrointestinal biopsies are also described. A final section briefly outlines immunohistochemical techniques in paraffin sections of formalin-fixed tissue. Immunohistochemistry is a static staining technique like any other histological staining (e.g. hemalum-eosin staining). It is less reliable than the enzyme histochemical technique.

It is the hope of the authors that the technical advice and the many pictures of characteristic anomalies in the gut may be helpful in the understanding and diagnosis of the different intestinal diseases which cause chronic constipation.

Preface

The first edition of the book on pathology of chronic constipation was drafted as an atlas folio. It enjoyed a brisk demand and sold out in the first year. This encouraged us to prepare the second edition 7 years later.

It has been demonstrated that enzyme histochemistry of native seromuscular intestinal biopsies allows the evaluation of nerve cell size and their dehydrogenase activity to recognize plexus immaturity in babies and inborn hypoplasia of the myenteric plexus in adults.

The acetylcholinesterase (AChE) activity of nerve fibers in circular and longitudinal muscles provides information about the motility performance of a particular intestinal part. This is important as it tells the surgeon whether an intestinal section is unable to transport its content properly, and it is a possible indication for resection in cases of negative findings. The nerve cell supply of the myenteric plexus and the parasympathetic tonus (AChE activity) of a proximal resection edge is a reliable source of information that the surgeon needs for a successful curative therapy.

Mucosa suction rectum biopsies offer a reliable diagnosis of an inborn aganglionosis (Hirschsprung's disease) by the pathological increased AChE activity in parasympathetic nerves of mucosa and muscularis mucosae.

The use of native seromuscular intestinal biopsies, cut in a cryostat, avoids shrinking artefacts in circular muscles of the intestinal wall as is usually observed in formalin-fixed tissue. Shrinking artefacts of circular muscles prevents the pathologist from recognizing the extension of an atrophy or myopathy in circular muscles.

The heretofore neglected tendinous collagen net in the muscularis propria and plexus layer, which operates intestinal peristalsis, provides information about its stenotic effect if this structure is atrophied by inflammation or X-ray lesion. Crohn's disease, diverticulitis, and ulcerative colitis destroy, via leukocytic collagenases, the tendinous net in muscularis propria and plexus layer, causing a stenotic symptomatology.

Architectural abnormalities of the muscularis propria as a doubling of the plexus layer explain focal stenotic symptoms. Smooth muscles myopathies are rare but serious reasons of an aperistaltic syndrome.

This book offers insights into many functional disturbances of intestinal motility, which are often not recognizable in formalin-fixed and standard HE-stained sections. It increases our diagnostic spectrum in chronic constipation. *Histopathology of Chronic Constipation* is an important reference book for pathologists in the diagnosis of chronic constipation; however, surgeons, gastroenterologists, and pediatricians will also find it important for understanding the reasons behind intestinal transport problems.

Acknowledgments

The authors are grateful to the staff of the Institute of Pathology of the University of Basel for their technical assistance.

Thanks go in particular to the technicians of the enzyme histochemical laboratory and the excellent work of Elisabeth Meier, Marlies Kasper, and Sabine Ipsen, all of whom made the book possible.

We sincerely thank Thomas Schürch of the photographic unit of the institute for the invaluable help in preparing and printing the illustrations.

Introduction

Chronic constipation is a fairly frustrating matter in classical histopathology as hemalum-eosin staining allows only a limited diagnostic statement. This, however, has changed in recent decades. Today, the foundation of histopathological diagnosis of gastrointestinal motility disorder is enzyme histochemistry. Many different gut diseases have been clearly diagnosed by enzyme histochemical techniques, such as Hirschsprung's disease (HD), ultrashort rectum aganglionosis, hypoganglionosis, immaturity of the enteral nervous system, intestinal neuronal dysplasia, and atrophic alterations of the lamina propria [1, 2].

Compared to enzyme histochemistry, immunohistochemistry in paraffin-embedded formalin-fixed tissue is presently only of limited value. The diagnosis of HD was a breakthrough for enzyme histochemistry. It is possible to diagnose HD reliably in rectum mucosa biopsies with the aid of an acetylcholinesterase reaction [3–5], which has become the gold standard in the diagnosis of HD [1, 6–8]. Today, enzyme histochemistry is the technique of choice in experimental pathology, as well as in the histopathological differential diagnosis of chronic constipation [9].

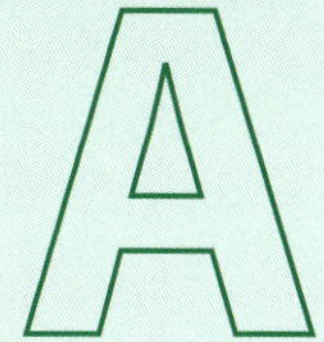

Histopathological Diagnosis

A.1

Enzyme Histochemical Differential Diagnosis in Chronic Constipation

When enzyme histochemistry is mentioned, the question arises: 'Why is HE (hemalum-eosin) staining in formalin-fixed tissue not enough?'

Enzyme histochemistry is a morphological technique which gives first-time functional information [9–12]. It is an important link to conventional histology, immunohistochemistry, and molecular pathology. It offers orthoptic localization of a particular enzyme in nerve cells and nerve fibers, as well as parenchymal cells, and reflects the metabolic rate of a particular cell by enzymes of the citric cycle. In contrast to other methods which only give static information, enzyme histochemistry is a sensitive and dynamic method which demonstrates a metabolic imbalance in pathological processes [9–12]. Enzyme histochemistry offers insights in the pathophysiology of HD and other diseases.

Figure 1 demonstrates in which way conventional histological staining relates to enzyme histochemistry.

Besides lactic dehydrogenase (LDH) and succinic dehydrogenase (SDH), which are used in the diagnosis of muscle biopsies, acetylcholinesterase (AChE) is routinely used in standard pathological laboratories as a key reaction in HD [13].

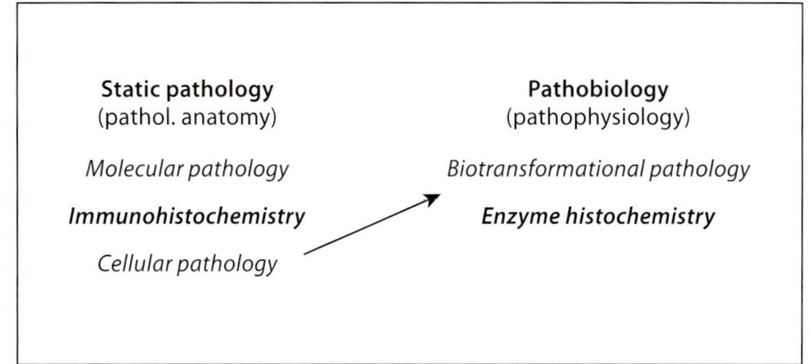

Fig. 1. Schematic representation of conventional staining (left) and enzyme histochemistry (right). Both techniques function complementarily. Conventional HE staining delineates the different tissue compartments and is a technique of static pathology. Enzyme histochemistry highlights functional alterations and elucidates the pathophysiology of a particular disease.

Rudolf Virchow postulated 160 years ago that the aim of pathological diagnostic research is the recognition of the pathophysiology of a particular disease [14, 15]. Enzyme histochemistry is the first morphologic method able to give insights into the pathophysiology of a particular disease [9, 16–18], and has proven to be the technique of choice in the diagnostic of gastrointestinal motility disorders [9, 18–21].

Functional Histopathological Differential Diagnosis in Colonic Motility Disorder

It has been demonstrated in recent years that a high number of different anomalies of the myenteric plexus or submucous plexus and smooth muscles of the lamina propria cause chronic constipation [2, 4, 13, 22].

Differential diagnosis of chronic constipation contains a high number of different diseases, which require different therapeutic strategies. These diseases include:

- HD
- Ultrashort HD
- Sphincter achalasia
- Total colonic aganglionosis
- Hypoganglionosis
- Immaturity of the enteral nervous system of mature babies
- Architectural malformation of the muscularis propria
- Atrophic alterations of the muscularis propria
- Intestinal neuronal dysplasia type A (NEC)
- Intestinal neuronal dysplasia type B
- Multiple endocrine neoplasia 2B
- Aplastic desmosis of the muscularis propria
- Atrophic desmosis of the muscularis propria
- Degenerative myopathy

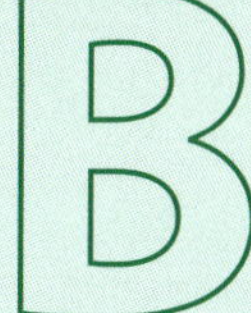

Different Colon Diseases with Chronic Constipation

Pathogenesis of Hirschsprung's Disease

Neuroblasts of the neck vagus migrate during embryonic weeks 6–12 craniocaudally along circular muscles to form a myenteric plexus. With a delay of several days, nerve cells of the myenteric plexus migrate into the submucosa to generate a submucous plexus.

During embryonic weeks 5–12, nerve fibers invade into circular muscles and mucosa of the distal colon from the sacral roots S2–S5. This happens 4 to 5 weeks before neuroblasts arrive in the descending colon. These nerves from the sacrum release acetylcholine in a synchronous manner. This causes a spastic contraction in the rectosigmoid up to the synaptic linking of these nerves with the invading neurocrest cells. This is a long-lasting process from embryonic weeks 10–12. It is a very sensitive period during which neuroblasts connect synaptic with parasympathetic nerves of sacral roots S2–S5. If neuroblasts do not arrive in the distal colon, HD or an aganglionosis develops. Therefore, HD is limited to the rectosigmoid or rectum in about 75% of babies.

In cases of rectum aganglionosis, nerve cells which modulate the permanent firing nerves from the sacral roots are missing, causing a spastic contraction of circular muscles and thus gut obstruction. Because acetylcholine and AChE have the same level, AChE can be used to evaluate the cholinergic level of a particular tissue. This fact is used in enzyme histochemistry to recognize an aganglionosis in the rectal mucosa. The increase of AChE activity in parasympathetic nerve fibers of the rectum mucosa can be used as a reliable indicator of an aganglionosis. AChE activity increases dependently with age (fig. 2–6). LDH and SDH or nitroxide synthase (NOS), which stain nerve cells electively, can be used as a second indicator of an aganglionosis (fig. 7).

Indicators of Hirschsprung's Disease

1 Increased acetylcholine release and AChE activity of parasympathetic nerves in lamina propria mucosae, muscularis mucosae, and muscularis propria are the result of an aganglionosis of the submucous and myenteric plexus (fig. 2–6).
2 A permanent release of acetylcholine by an inborn aganglionosis causes a spasticity of the muscularis propria in the distal colon.
3 The aganglionic segment of the rectum or rectosigmoid causes an obstruction in the distal colon.

Immaturity of nerve cells, often observed in young babies, show low SDH and LDH activity in nerve cells. In these cases, an unspecific reaction of NOS or NADH diaphorase may be helpful to establish aganglionosis of the submucosa. It is a great advantage to use only mucosa bi-

Fig. 2. a HD. Characteristic increase of AChE in parasympathetic nerve fibers of lamina propria mucosae and muscularis mucosae (2-week-old boy; compare with fig. 97). **b** Normal innervated rectum mucosa; 4-week-old boy. AChE staining. ×45.

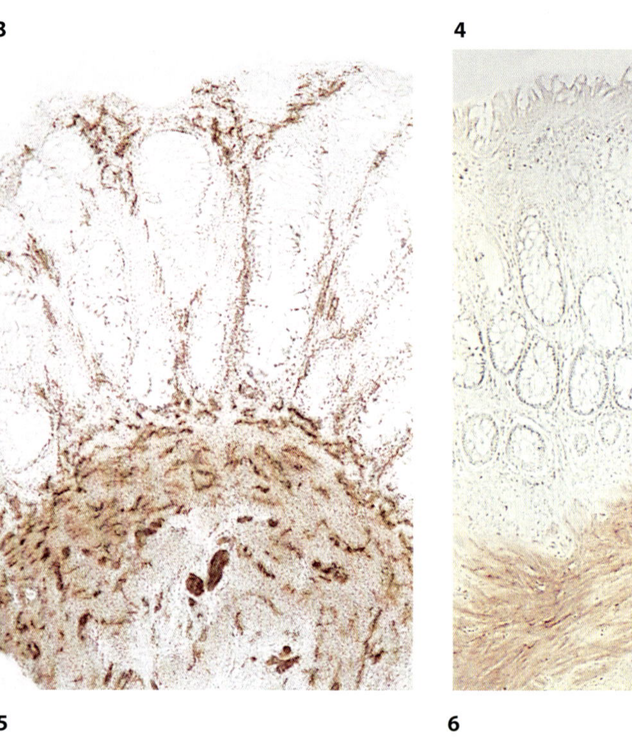

Fig. 3. Mucosa biopsy from the rectum (native cryostat section) with characteristic increase of AChE activity in parasympathetic nerve fibers in muscularis mucosae and lamina propria mucosae: HD. AChE reaction without counterstaining. ×90.

Fig. 4. AChE reaction of normal innervated rectum mucosa (native cryostat section). Only in muscularis mucosae are weakly stained nerve fibers to be observed. ×90.

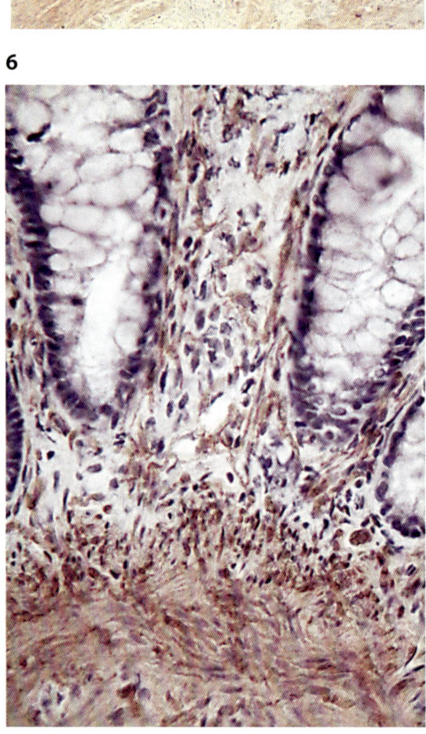

Fig. 5. Higher magnification of aganglionic mucosa biopsy section without counterstaining (7-month-old boy). ×180.

Fig. 6. Aganglionic rectum mucosa as in figure 5 with hemalum counterstaining. The identification of increased AChE activity in nerve fibers is much more difficult than in figure 5 without counterstaining. ×180.

Histopathology of Chronic Constipation

opsies for HD diagnosis, thus avoiding anesthesia for a whole-mount biopsy or a laparoscopic seromuscular biopsy of the sigmoid [4, 13, 20, 23, 24].

In order not to miss a distal aganglionosis, the first biopsy may be taken from the rectoanal transition. Biopsies which are taken proximal from the anal ring may be taken in geometric distances (2, 4, and 8 cm above the anal ring). A seromuscular biopsy of the sigmoid allows no exclusion of an aganglionosis in the distal rectum [25, 26].

An enzyme histochemical AChE reaction in native rectal mucosa biopsy sections is considered to be the gold standard in the diagnosis of HD. This was proven as 100% reliable after 20–30 years of diagnostic experience [2, 20, 23, 27–30].

The advantage of the AChE reaction is that there is only the need to look for nerve fibers with increased enzyme activity and not for nerve cells of submucous plexus, which can be difficult if the enteric nervous system is immature or the submucosa was not biopsied [22, 31].

Diagnostic Criteria of Hirschprung's Disease

1 Increased AChE activity of parasympathetic nerve fibers in the rectal mucosa and muscularis mucosae (fig. 2–6).
2 Aganglionosis of the submucous and myenteric plexus (fig. 7).
3 Diagnostic criteria are limited to the rectum and rectosigmoid.

The characteristics of increased AChE activity in nerve fibers of lamina propria mucosae and circular muscles of the lamina propria are limited to the distal part of the colon in HD by embryological reasons (fig. 8, 9). Nerve fiber density shows in aganglionic colon in the distal colon a decrease in the caudocranial direction (fig. 10) [13].

It should be mentioned that AChE activity in parasympathetic nerve fibers increases with the age of the baby in HD [32]. This is, however, of minor importance if the cryostat sections are at least 12- to 15-μm thick and have an end-thickness of 3.6–4.5 μm after spreading and drying on a microscopic slide [33].

It is also important to stain LDH, SDH, and NOS to evaluate nerve cells. This serves as second proof of an aganglionosis. NOS or NADH diaphorase is particularly helpful as it identifies immature nerve cells which have a low SDH (and LDH) activity.

The aim of intraoperative examination of HD is to recognize if the proximal resection line is still aganglionic, hypoganglionic, or normal innervated. A NOS or NADH reaction is particularly helpful to stain nerve cells. A rapid AChE reaction [34–37] is not very helpful because the progressive caudocranial decrease of nerve fiber density, as mentioned above, has the risk that a negative rapid AChE reaction may indicate a normal innervation of the proximal resection ring.

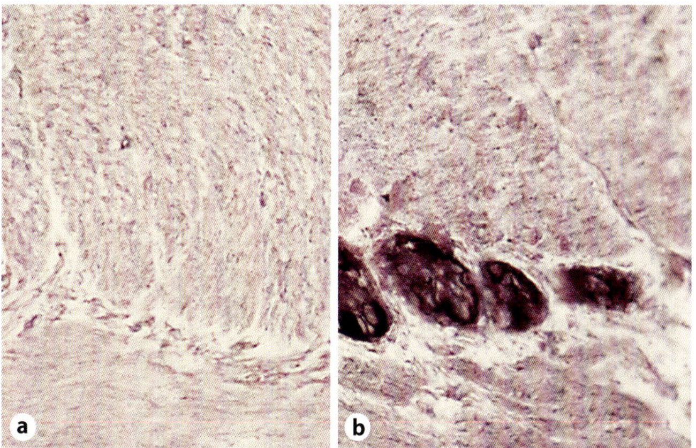

Fig. 7. Comparison of aganglionic (**a**) and ganglion-containing (**b**) myenteric plexus in an LDH reaction. ×240.

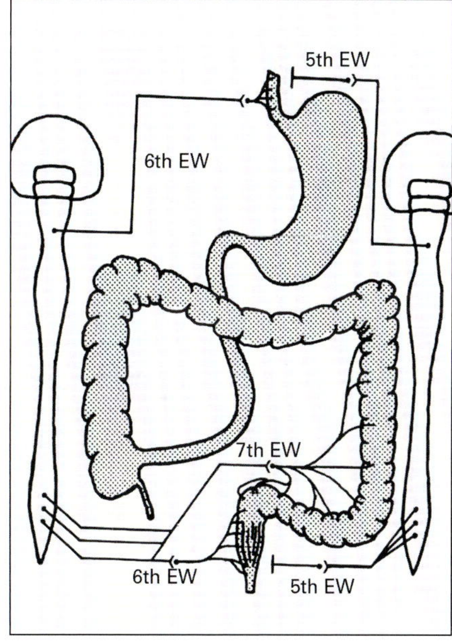

Fig. 8. Schematic representation of the embryology of the parasympathetic nerves from the sacral roots S2–S4. The extramural innervation of the distal colon develops during embryonic weeks (EW) 5–7.

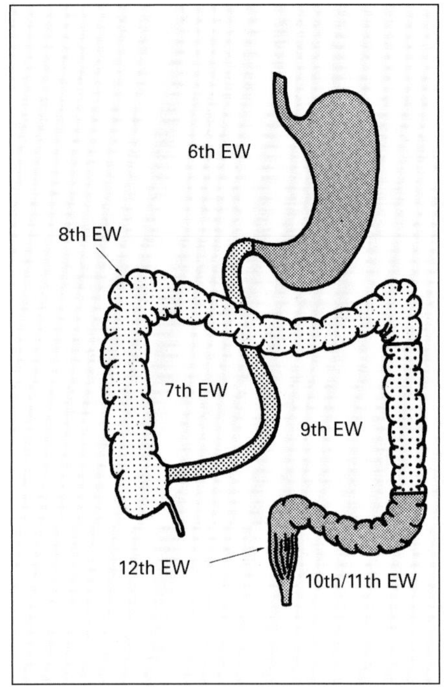

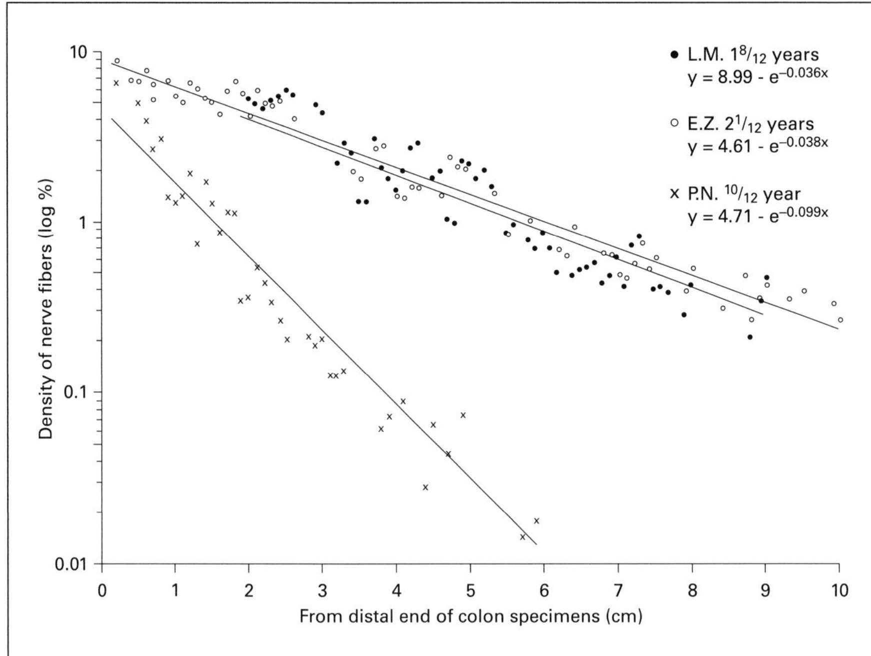

Fig. 9. Schematic drawing of the embryological colonization of the gut by neuroblasts from the neck vagus, which arrive at the distal colon during EW 9–12.

Fig. 10. Morphometric measurements of nerve fiber density in circular muscles of total colonic aganglionosis showing an exponential caudocranial decrease. The steeper curve (bottom) is typical for a hypoplastic extramural parasympathetic innervation of circular muscles.

In formalin-fixed paraffin-embedded tissue, immunohistochemical calretinin reaction can be used. The absence of nerve fibers in the rectum mucosa is an important characteristic for the diagnosis of HD [38].

Incidence of Hirschsprung's Disease

Sixty to seventy percent of children with HD have an isolated aganglionosis in the distal colon [5, 39, 40]. Ten to twenty percent have an aganglionosis up to the splenic flexure. Only 3–6% show a total colon aganglionosis [41–43].

Ten to twenty-three percent of children with trisomy 21 suffer from HD, the incidence rate of which is 5 times higher in boys than in girls. The risk of developing HD is in brothers of sisters with aganglionosis 18% higher than in sisters of brothers (2%).

Genetic Approach of Hirschsprung's Disease

HD is a genetically heterogeneous disease. Ten percent of HD patients show genetic defects in other organs in addition to aganglionosis.

The most important gene in the development of HD is a receptor tyrosine kinase (RET). HD is a neurocristopathy characterized by a disturbed immigration of neuroblasts into the rectosigmoid or the whole colon [39]. Further genetic studies have shown that gene alterations are disease-causing mutations [44, 45], and recent studies have demonstrated that 8–10 genes are involved in this neurocristopathy [40, 46–49]. The RET gene has proven to be the major gene in the etiology of HD [43, 50, 51]. However, only 20% of RET mutations develop HD [52].

A series of rare congenital disorders are linked with Hirschsprung's syndrome. The Waardenberg or Shaw-Waardenberg syndrome is associated with mutations of the Sox 10 gene [53–55]. It was demonstrated that neuronal crest cells and glia cells of the peripheral nervous system express Sox 10 [56, 57]. In 1998, Mowat-Wilson syndrome was described, which is combined with HD [58]. In rare cases, Mowat-Wilson syndrome is associated with congenital heart failure [59]. Chondrodysplasia syndrome or the cartilage-hair hypoplasia is a seldom observed syndrome which can accompany HD [60, 61]. Down syndrome is frequently linked to HD.

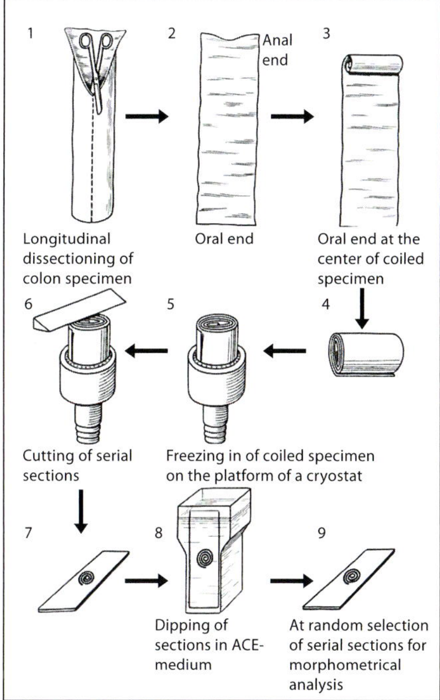

Fig. 11. Schematic representation of cutting and histochemical processing of a coiled colon specimen with an aganglionosis.

B.2

'Swiss-Roll Technique'

The 'Swiss-Roll Technique' owes its name to our laboratory rolling (caudocranial) operative gut specimens (15 cm long × 2 cm broad stripes) so as to get an overview of the whole specimen [62–64].

The advantage of this procedure is to measure the exact length of the aganglionic segment, the extension of hypoganglionosis proximal of aganglionosis, and the length of the proximal normal innervated gut (fig. 11, 12). This preparation is an ideal prerequisite for a morphometric quantification of the myenteric plexus along the extension of the resected gut specimen.

An important step for standardizing this technique was to measure the thickness of the cryostat section after spreading and drying on a microscopic slide. In addition, with a scanning microscope we visualized the section and compared it with a freeze-dried cryostat section. We demonstrated that by spreading and drying on a microscopic slide, a 15-μm thick cryostat section loses at least 70% of its thickness. With this treatment, the slide has an end-thickness of about 4 μm, which is compatible to a paraffin section [65].

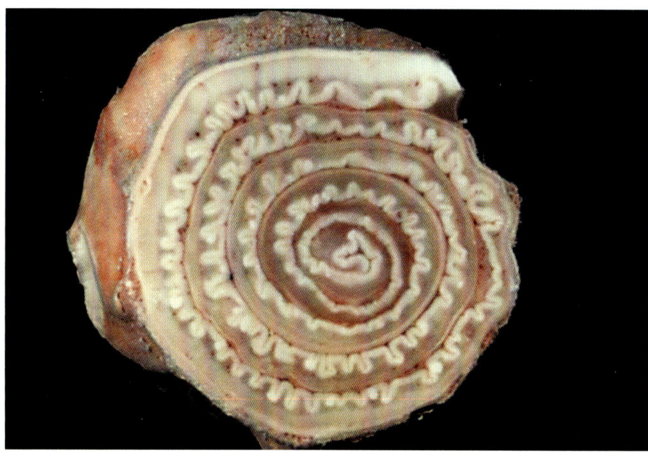

Fig. 12. Caudocranially coiled surgical specimen (Swiss roll) on a cryostat carrier.

We observed in such Swiss-roll preparations that a hypoganglionic segment proximal of an aganglionosis has a 50% decrease of nerve cells per millimeter length of colon. Ganglion distances of the myenteric plexus are doubled [66, 67]. All morphometric measurements were performed with optic electronic semiautomatic cell analysis equipment (ASBA 3; Wild and Leitz Co.). Nerve cells and ganglia of the myenteric plexus were stained with a LDH or NOS reaction which discriminates significantly nerve cells and myenteric plexus against surrounding tissue. With this particular technique, it is possible for the clinician to ascertain the length of the resected aganglionosis and hypoganglionosis (fig. 13).

The Swiss-roll technique is performed as follows (fig. 11):

1 The resected gut specimen is prepared free of fat tissue.
2 The specimen is cut open.
3 In the proximal and distal resection line, a 2-cm-long part transversal to the length of the resected gut specimen is prepared and cryostat cut.
4 The opened gut is spread on filter paper with mucosa on the side of the paper.
5 The gut is divided in 10- to 15-cm-long parts.
6 A 2-cm-broad strip is prepared from each part and caudocranially rolled with two surgical pincers; mucosa must be outside.
7 Each role is fixed with Tissue-Teck® or white of egg on a cryostat tissue carrier and frozen on a bed of CO_2 granulate (–80°C)

Fig. 13. Representation of a morphometric ganglion measurement proximal to an aganglionosis (HD) [66]. The first part (distal) represents a hypoplastic dysganglionosis. In the middle, a hypoganglionic segment is shown. The proximal part is characteristic of a normal myenteric plexus (single ganglion measurement by an optic-electronic image analysis system). LDH stained section.

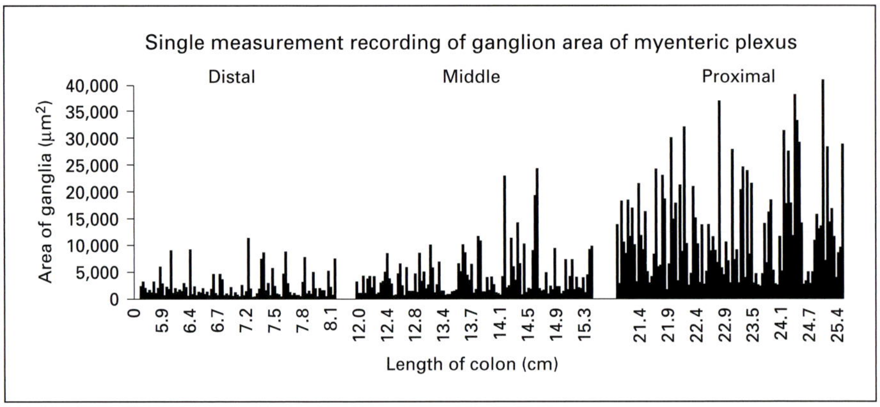

B.3

Intraoperative Evaluation of the Myenteric Plexus

The aim of an evaluation of the myenteric plexus in the proximal resection line is to be able to recognize a hypoganglionosis intraoperatively (fig. 13). From a clinical point of view, the aim of this procedure is to avoid recidivation of an occlusive syndrome or chronic constipation [68–71]. Whole-mount biopsies taken intraoperatively were cut on a cryostat and incubated for a NADH diaphorase reaction. This had the advantage of being able to evaluate an immature, hypoganglionic, or normal innervated myenteric plexus after an incubation time of 5–8 min.

The reliability of this diagnosis depends on the size of the whole-mount biopsies sent for diagnosis. It may be helpful to have 3–4 seromuscular biopsies, taken every 2 cm proximal to the resection line.

B.4

Ultrashort Hirschsprung's Disease

Ultrashort HD can be reliably diagnosed in the first centimeters of the rectum by an increased AChE reaction in nerve fibers of the muscularis mucosa and submucosa. The histochemical picture is different from classical HD because no or extremely few AChE-positive nerve fibers are observed in lamina propria mucosae (fig. 14–16).

Some cases are limited to the anal ring and show nerve fibers with increased AChE activity in the musculus corrugator cutis ani, the most distal part of the internal sphincter (fig. 17, 18).

Characteristics of Ultrashort Hirschsprung's Disease [4]

1 AChE-positive nerve fibers in muscularis mucosae, submucosa and musculus corrugator cutis ani (fig. 14, 16, 17).
2 Missing nets of AChE-positive nerve fibers in lamina propria mucosae (fig. 14–16).
3 Start of obstruction symptomatology with ending of weaning.

Ultrashort HD causes outlet constipation, and it is only sporadically observed between 4 and 30 years of age [72, 73]. A reliable diagnosis of ultrashort HD can be made exclusively with an AChE reaction [74–76]. Because ultrashort HD ends at 4 cm, it is important to have a normal colon mucosa biopsy 5 cm above the dentate line. The 5- to 6-cm biopsy is so important because in rare cases total colon aganglionosis with a hypoplasia of the extramural parasympathetic innervation still shows characteristics of ultrashort HD which indicate a long aganglionic segment in the 5-cm biopsy.

Forms of Ultrashort Hirschsprung's Disease [4]

1 Aganglionosis extending 3–4 cm above anal ring.
2 Aganglionosis of the anal ring.
3 Aganglionosis of the musculus corrugator cutis ani (fig. 17, 18).

A cautious sphincter dilatation by means of Hegar Boogies or a manual dilatation may often be sufficient to compensate outlet constipation [77]. If manual dilatation is not successful, an anorectal posterior myectomy is recommended [78, 79]. Better therapeutic strategies may be developed once ultrashort HD can be more reliably diagnosed.

Histopathology of Chronic Constipation

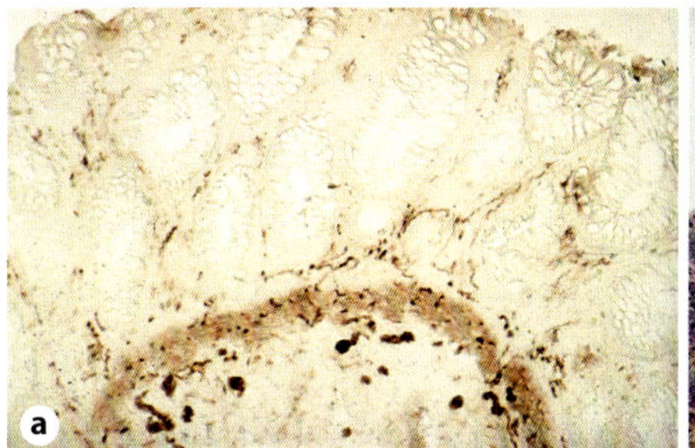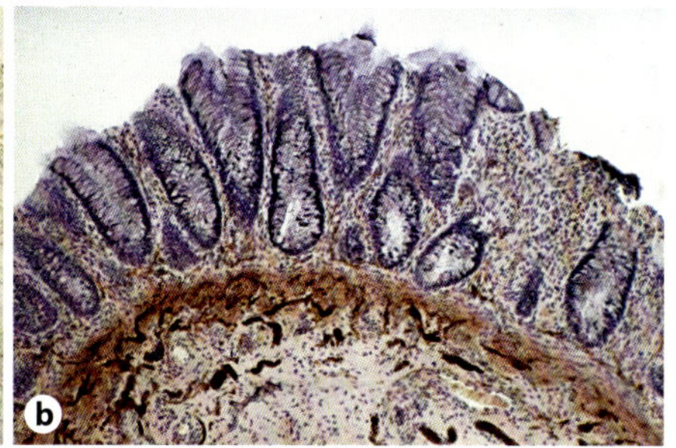

Fig. 14. a Ultrashort HD 3 cm above the anal ring with characteristic increase of AChE in nerves of muscularis mucosae and big nerve fibers in the submucosa. In contrast to normal HD, rarely developed nerve fibers in the lamina propria mucosae can be observed. **b** Same section with hemalum counterstaining. ×90.

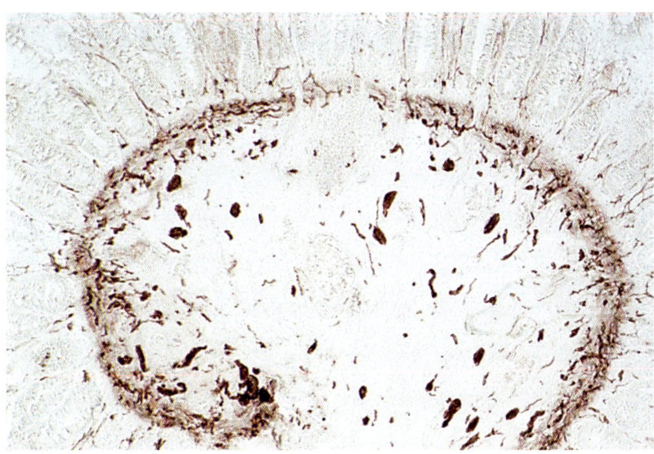

Fig. 15. Ultrashort HD with characteristic increase of AChE activity in nerve fibers of the muscularis mucosae and submucosa [73]. ×75.

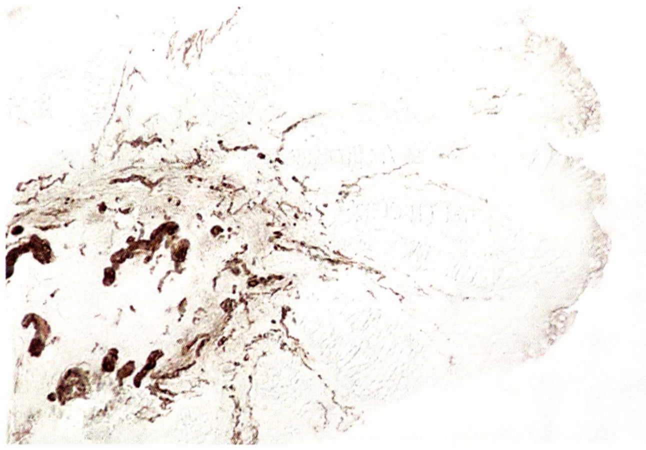

Fig. 16. Ultrashort HD with increased AChE activity in nerve fibers of the muscularis mucosae and afferent nerves in the submucosa. ×120.

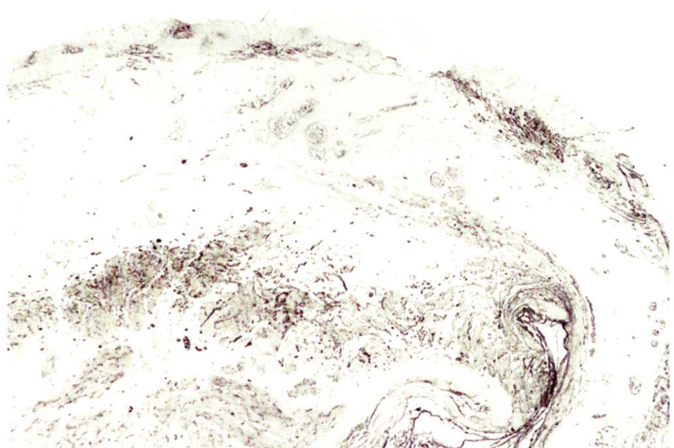

Fig. 17. Increase of AChE activity in nerve fibers of aganglionic musculus corrugator cutis ani in the rectoanal transitional zone. ×120.

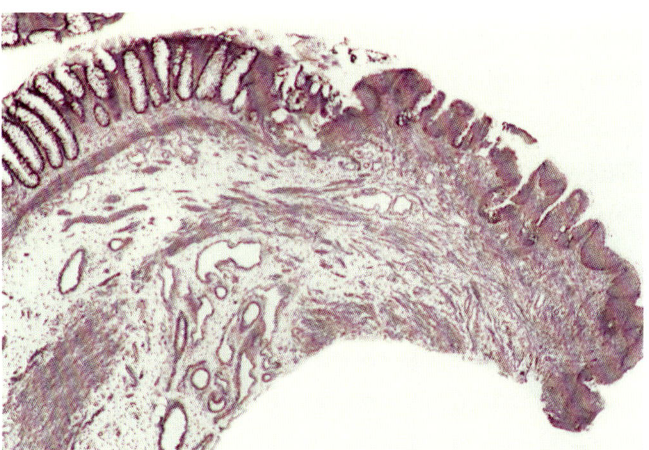

Fig. 18. Insertion of musculus corrugator cutis ani in the transition from muscularis mucosae to anal skin. LDH reaction. ×75.

Total Aganglionosis of the Colon

Mucosa biopsies of the rectum and sigmoid, descending, transverse, and ascending colon may demonstrate a total aganglionosis of the colon. Rectal and sigmoid mucosa biopsies normally show increased AChE activity in parasympathic nerve fibers like classical HD. Due to anatomical reasons, no AChE-positive structures can be observed in the mucosa of the transverse and ascending colon. At this stage, it is helpful to take laparoscopic seromuscular biopsies from the transverse and ascending colon and terminal ileum so as to define the length of the aganglionosis. Additionally, the AChE reaction may also be in LDH and NOS reactions, proving aganglionosis of the myenteric plexus [79]. It may be favorable to coil a caudocranially resected specimen (fig. 19, 20) to get an overview of the total length of the resected gut (fig. 11; see section on Swiss-Roll Technique). It becomes obvious that nerve fiber density with increased AChE activity in the aganglionic segment of the distal colon decreases in the caudocranial direction from the rectum to the descending colon (fig. 21–24) [42, 64]. This allows objectifying the extension of the extramural parasympathetic innervation from the sacral roots (fig. 21, 22). In total aganglionosis, proliferation of sacral parasympathetic nerves is often retarded or hypoplastic (fig. 20).

Recently, total intestinal aganglionosis has been treated with gut transplantation [80, 81] with a survival rate of about 62%. Long-term examinations (up to 30 years) after resecting aganglionic colon have shown that long-term outcome of these patients is quite favorable [42, 82–86].

The best surgical procedure in total aganglionosis (Soave or Martin procedure) is presently under discussion [84, 87]. Traditional surgery of total aganglionosis of the colon with ileorectostomy has shown an improvement of anorectal function over time.

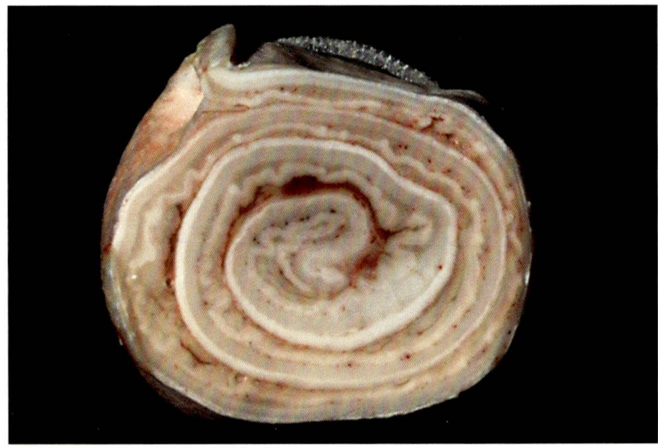

Fig. 19. Caudocranially coiled aganglionic colon (Swiss roll) on a cryostat carrier.

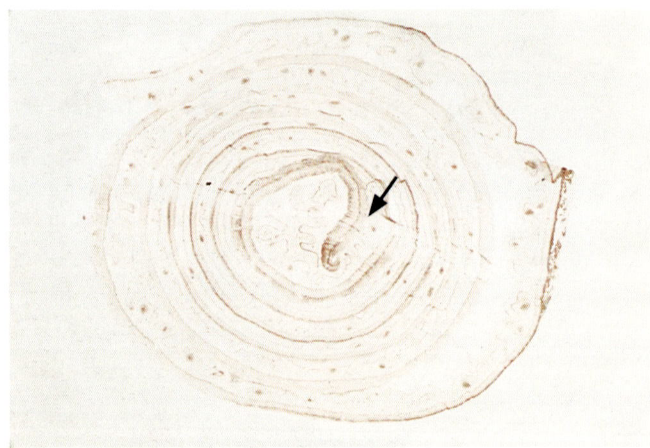

Fig. 20. Section of a coiled colon with total aganglionosis, showing the distal increase of AChE activity in the center (arrow). Due to anatomical reasons (see fig. 8–10), the characteristics of HD are limited to the rectosigmoid.

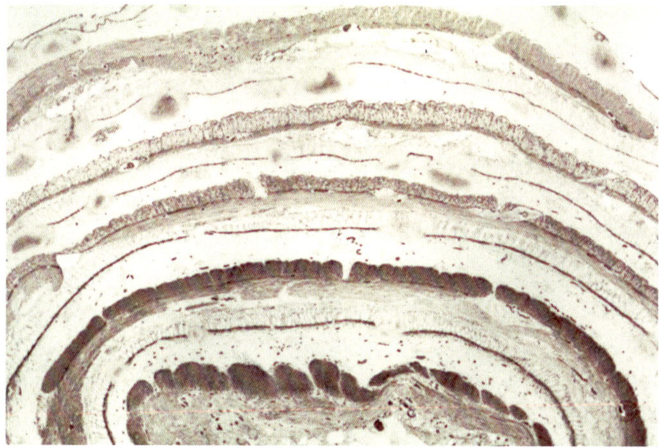

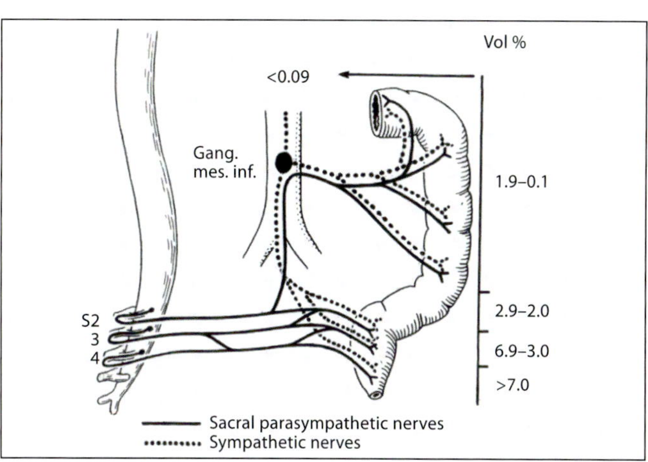

Fig. 21. Magnification of a coiled surgical specimen with total aganglionosis. The four layers of the coiled aganglionic colon show the caudocranial decrease of AChE-containing nerve fibers (compare with fig. 8–10). ×18.

Fig. 22. Schematic representation of the nerve fiber density in circular muscles of total aganglionosis. The innervation of the distal colon arises from the sacral roots S2–S5 and ends in the proximal descending colon.

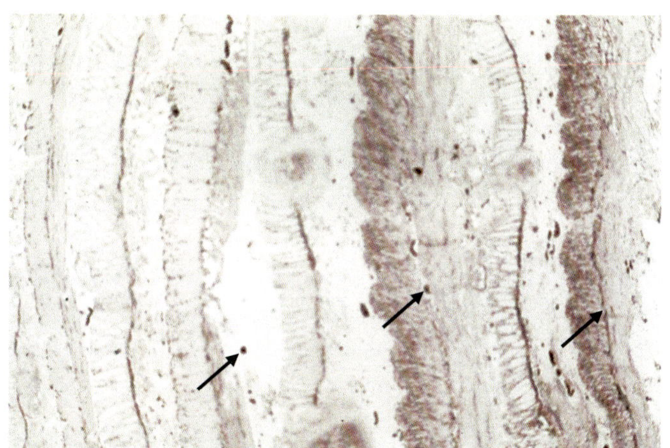

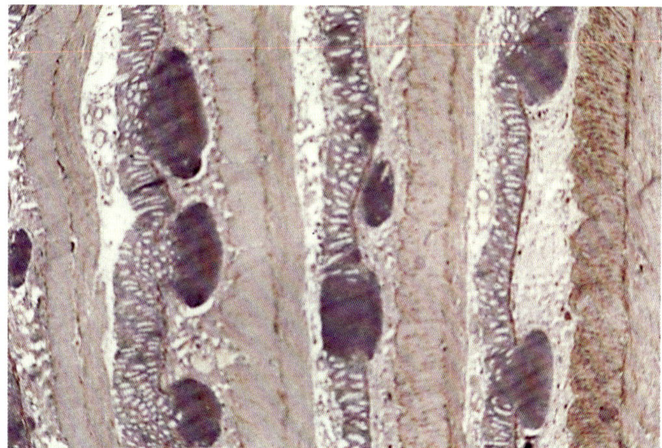

Fig. 23. Identical tissue as in figure 21. The aganglionosis of the myenteric plexus can be clearly recognized (arrows). The increase of nerve fiber density in the circular muscles of the distal colon is only obvious in the two right layers. ×36.

Fig. 24. Same section as in figure 23, but with hemalum counterstaining. ×36.

Hypoganglionosis of the myenteric plexus is a frequently observed anomaly in slow-transit constipation. This is reflected in the high number of publications referring to hypoganglionosis.

There are different forms of hypoganglionosis diagnosed in seromuscular biopsies: inborn hypoplastic dysganglionic hypoganglionosis (fig. 25, 26), oligoneuronal hypoganglionosis (often observed proximal of an aganglionic distal colon segment (fig. 27, 28)), and atrophic hypoganglionosis in adulthood (fig. 29, 30).

All these forms are characterized by slow-transit constipation and cannot be clinically objectified. The hypoplastic dysganglionic hypoganglionosis is often called pseudo-Hirschsprung. It is an important task for the pathologist to prove during the resection of an aganglionosis that the proximal resection edge is not hypoganglionic but normal innervated [66, 71, 88, 90–94]. The most feasible technique is a NOS or NADH diaphorase reaction to examine the myenteric plexus, which needs just 8–10 min of reaction time.

A diagnostic objectification of hypoganglionosis requires a collection of full-thickness or seromuscular biopsies from the rectum or sigmoid. Mucosa specimens of the rectum or sigmoid are not suitable for proving hypoganglionosis [95–99].

The diagnosis of hypoganglionosis used to be made mainly in a descriptive manner [2, 95, 100, 101]. In 1978, Munakata et al. [100] presented for the first time quantitative data about the number of ganglia, plexus area, and diameter of ganglia of the transitional area between the aganglionosis and normal innervated colon. These results were generated from horizontal sections and cannot be directly compared with data related to length (mm) of transverse cut sections of the colonic wall. Other quantitative morphometric measurements [89, 96, 102, 103] of the proximal margin of resected colons with HD have demonstrated values which cannot be directly compared with each other because of different staining techniques [104].

Morphometric results depend remarkably on the techniques used. Measurements from single cases show a high variation of ganglion area of the myenteric plexus in the transitional zone ranging from aganglionosis to regular innervated colon (fig. 13). However, all morphometric data, generated in different laboratories with different techniques, demonstrate identical trends: an increase of

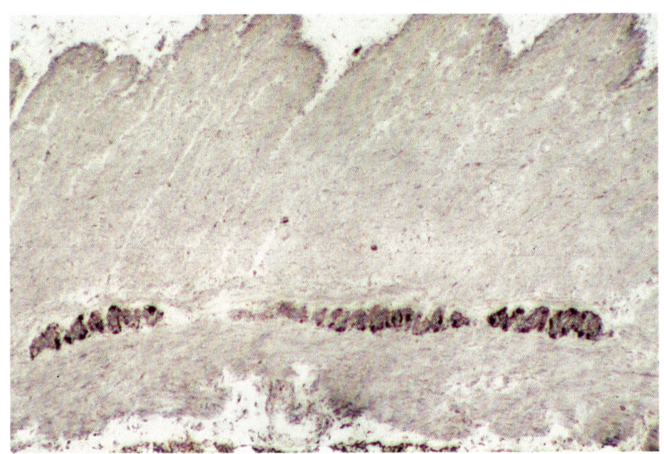

Fig. 25. Normal myenteric plexus. LDH. ×180.

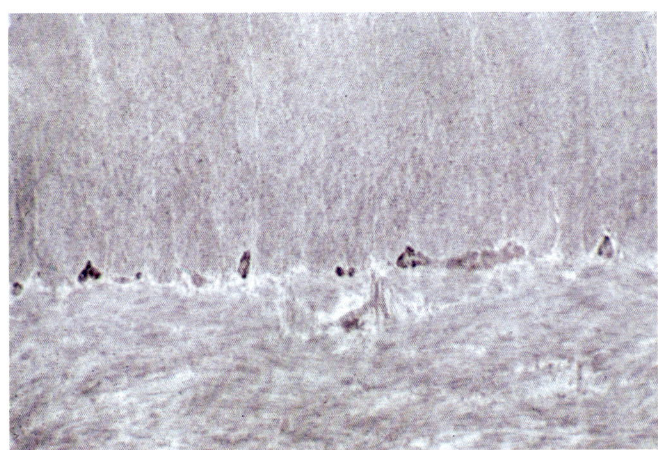

Fig. 26. Hypoplastic hypoganglionosis of the colon (compare with fig. 25). LDH reaction. ×180.

ganglion distances and a decrease of ganglion area, which is characteristic for the transitional zone between the distal aganglionic segment and normal innervated colon (fig. 13). The most important morphometric criteria for the diagnosis of a colonic hypoganglionosis are a 50% lower myenteric plexus area and nerve cell number. A further important parameter of a hypoplastic hypoganglionosis is the increase of ganglion distances [66, 67, 105].

The slow-transit constipation of a hypoganglionosis is accompanied by low cholinergic nerve activity [106, 107] in the muscularis propria.

A risk of chronic constipation by hypoganglionosis is the development of ischemic lesions in circular and longitudinal muscles of muscularis propria (fig. 31–35). The

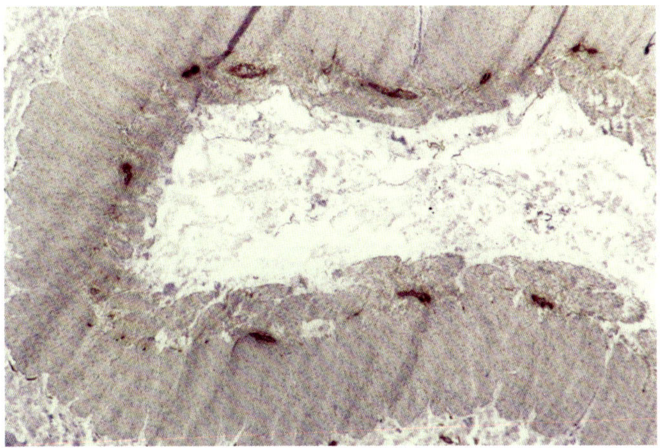

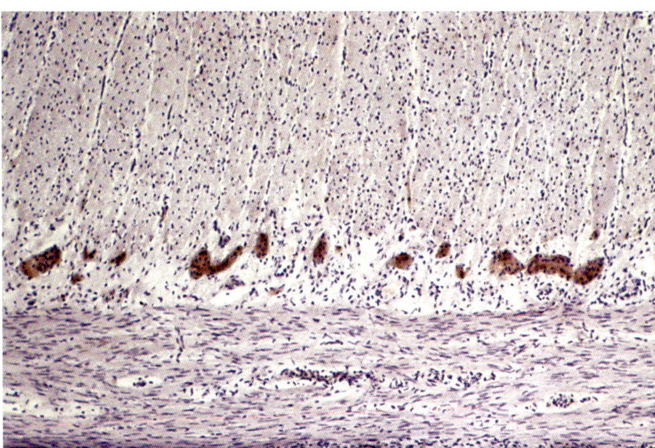

Fig. 27. Hypoplastic myenteric plexus. Moderately developed myenteric plexus with decreased nerve cell content (compare with fig. 28). The low AChE activity in nerve fibers of the muscularis propria represents the missing motility. AChE reaction without counterstaining. ×30.

Fig. 29. Normal myenteric plexus. AChE with hemalum counterstaining. ×180.

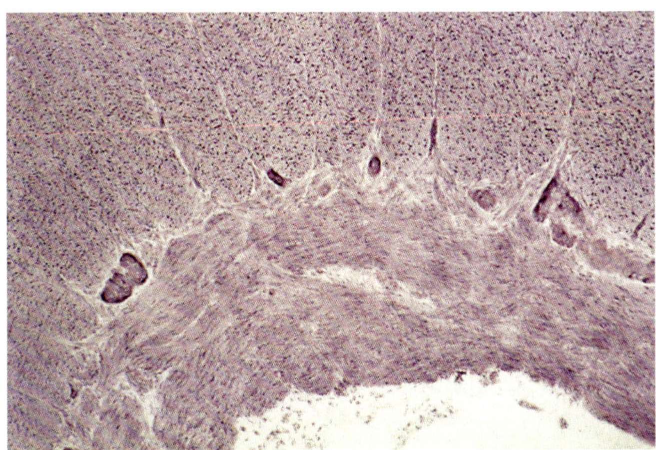

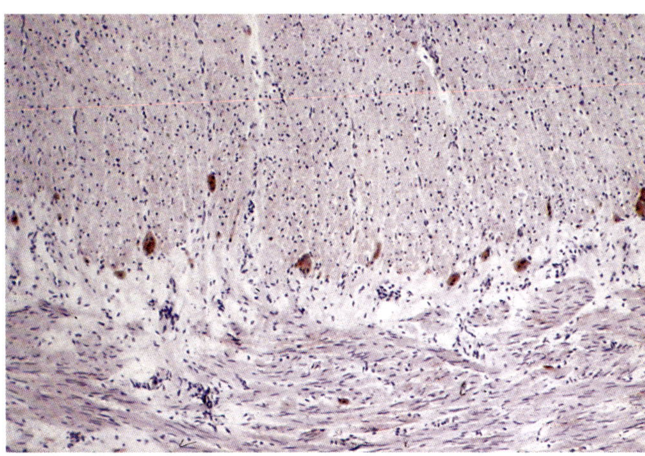

Fig. 28. Oligoneuronal hypoganglionosis. Immaturity of the enteric nervous system. Tiny nerve cells with low dehydrogenase activity are characteristic findings. LDH. ×30.

Fig. 30. Atrophic hypoganglionosis of myenteric plexus (compare with fig. 29). AChE. ×180.

consequence of ischemic lesions in smooth muscles of the colonic wall is scar formation and atrophy of the tendinous net in longitudinal and circular muscles which causes peristalsis of the colon [108]. Therefore, hypoganglionosis causes a progressive decline of colon transport performance. This can be avoided if hypoganglionosis of the colon is verified by laparoscopic seromuscular biopsies in childhood and consequently treated by resection of the hypoganglionic part of the colon, which is generally limited to the descending colon [90, 99, 109–111]. Under normal conditions, the most demanding transport performance takes place in the descending colon.

With reference to the pathogenesis of an atrophic hypoganglionosis, disturbed generation of trophic factors by glial cells of the myenteric plexus seems to be important [112–114]. A lack of the growth factors TRK-C and NT-3 may be involved in the development of a hypoganglionosis [115].

Atrophic hypoganglionosis is often observed in adults. It is characterized by a decrease of nerve cell number, nerve cell size, and low AChE activity [116]. It is an open question whether atrophic hypoganglionosis develops from a hypoplastic hypoganglionosis in childhood [115].

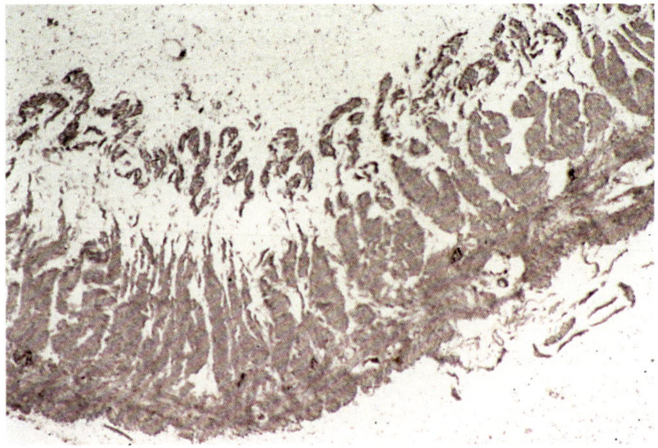

Fig. 31. Hypoganglionosis with ischemic atrophy of circular muscles. LDH reaction. ×64.

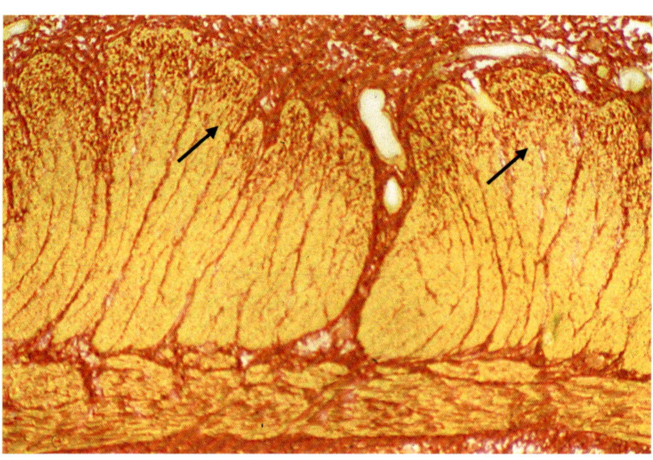

Fig. 34. Pricrosirius red staining of figure 33. Scar development in the inner layer of circular muscles (arrows; section angle 45°). ×64.

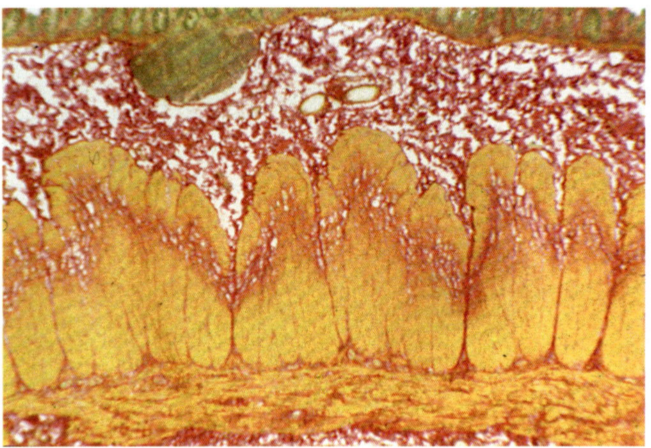

Fig. 32. Hypoganglionosis with ischemic scar formation in circular muscles. Picrosirius red staining. ×64.

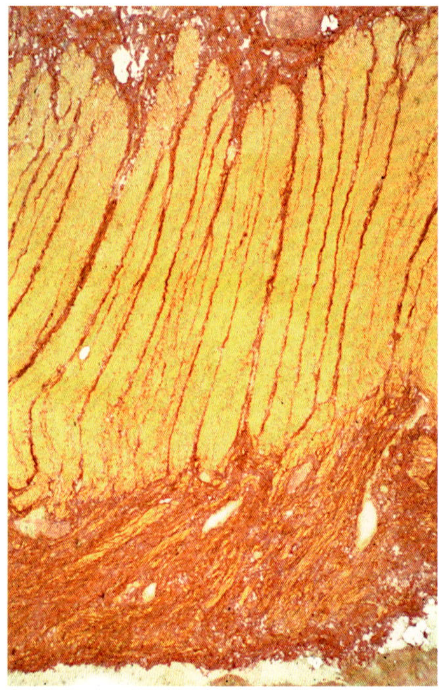

Fig. 35. Scar formation of longitudinal muscles in long-lasting hypoganglionosis. Picrosirius red staining. ×120.

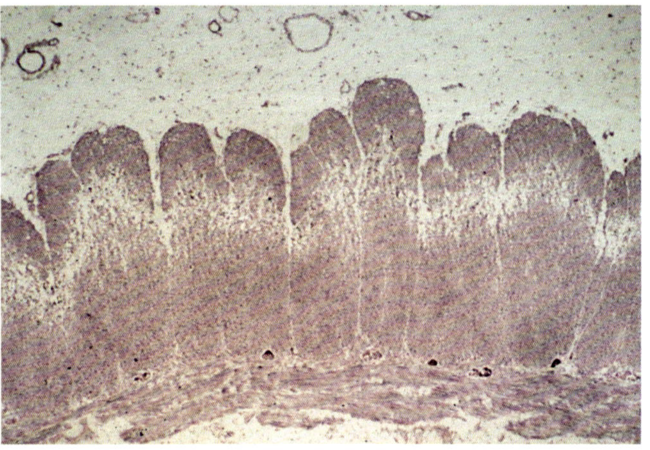

Fig. 33. Ischemic atrophy of circular muscles in hypoganglionosis of the myenteric plexus. LDH reaction. ×64.

Histopathology of Chronic Constipation

Immaturity of the Enteric Nervous System in Childhood

Only a few papers have investigated neuronal immaturity in the mature colon of young children. Several investigations have stressed the fact that a recurrence of chronic constipation after the resection of an aganglionic rectum is not always caused by hypoganglionosis, but rather by immaturity of the enteric nervous system [117–121].

Immaturity of the submucous and myenteric plexus is characterized by a faint reaction of mitochondrial enzyme activity (fig. 36–41). Immature nerve cells have low SDH activity (mitochondrial enzyme), which contrasts with the high activity of NADH diaphorase [122]. This immaturity can also be observed in mature babies without HD. It is important to be aware that an immature enteric nervous system in a mature baby needs 3 to 4 years to normalize. Trophic factors may mature the submucous and myenteric plexus [123] and increase SDH activity to the same level as NADH diaphorase and LDH activity. Immature nerve cells are very small and contrast clearly with mature nerve cells (fig. 42).

Nerve cell maturation in a premature baby normalizes parallel to the maturation of the baby in a few weeks. The maturation process can be followed in mucosal biopsies. No surgical intervention is necessary.

In some cases hypoganglionosis is combined with nerve cell immaturity. It is often difficult to differentiate between nerve cells and glia cells in immature ganglia [22, 88].

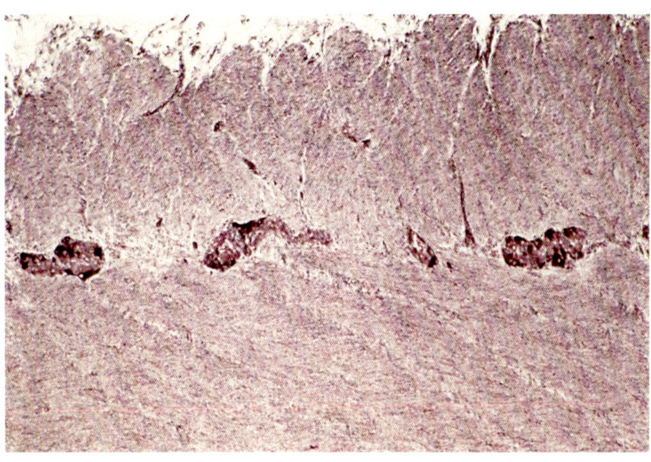

Fig. 36. Mature myenteric plexus with dehydrogenase-rich nerve cells. SDH reaction. ×75.

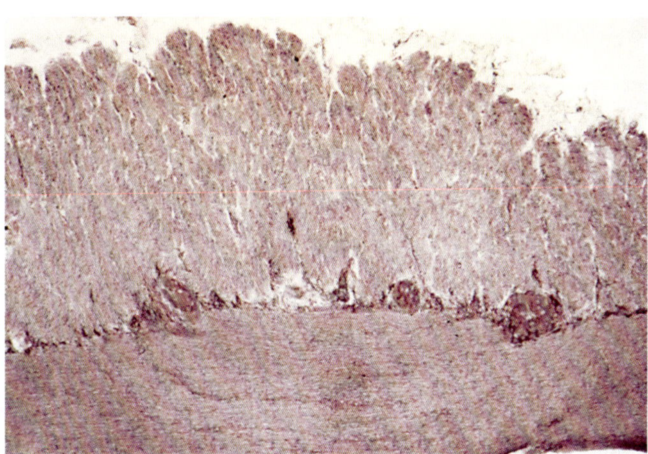

Fig. 37. Immaturity of myenteric plexus. Only few SDH-positive nerve cells can be recognized (12-month-old girl; compare with fig. 36). ×75.

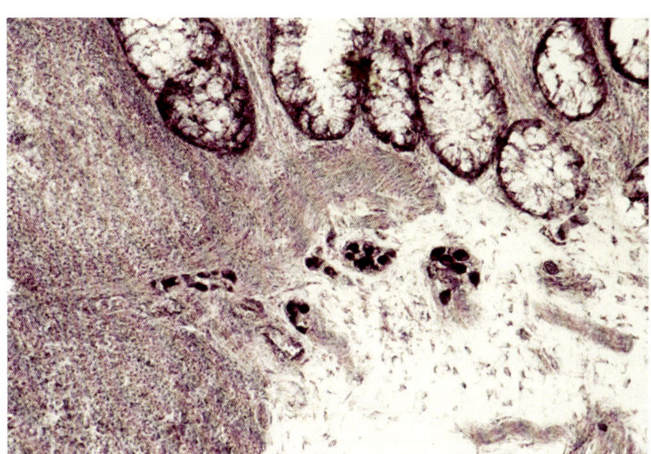

Fig. 38. Mature submucous plexus in a 1-month-old baby. SDH reaction. ×180.

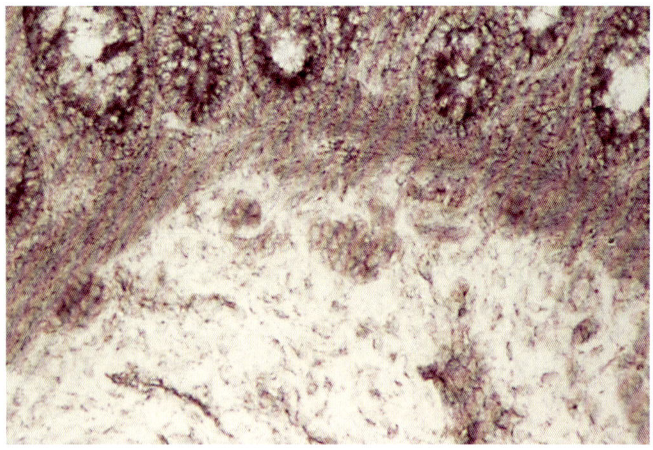

Fig. 39. Immature mucosa-biopsy of a 2-month-old girl. Only few SDH-positive nerve cells can be identified in ganglia of submucous plexus (compare with fig. 38). ×180.

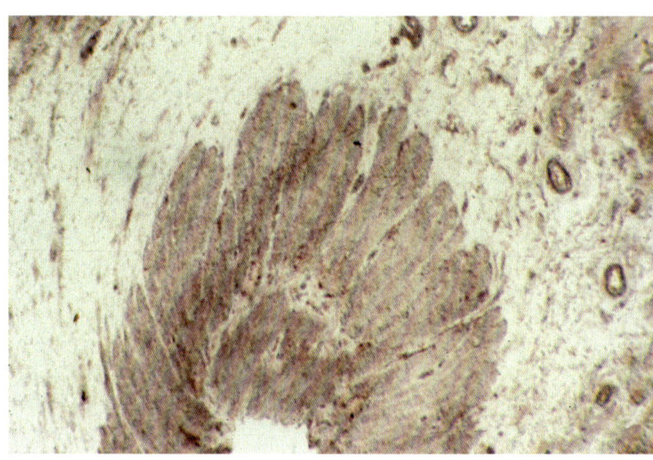

Fig. 41. Immature myenteric plexus in an SDH reaction. No nerve cells with a positive SDH reaction can be observed (compare with fig. 40). ×75.

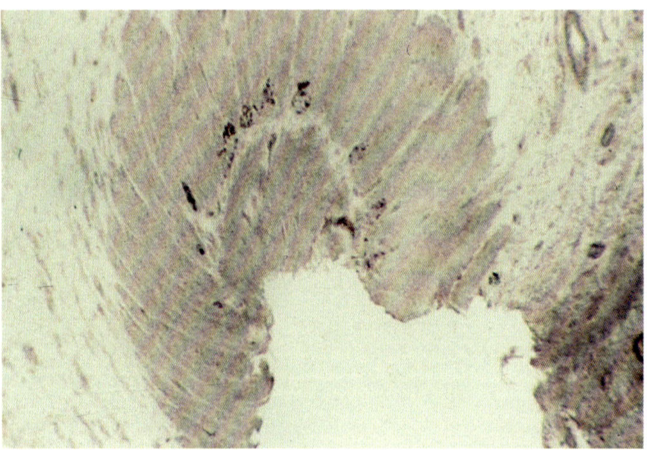

Fig. 40. Immature myenteric plexus in a NADPH diaphorase (NOS) reaction. The small nerve cells can be clearly recognized. ×75.

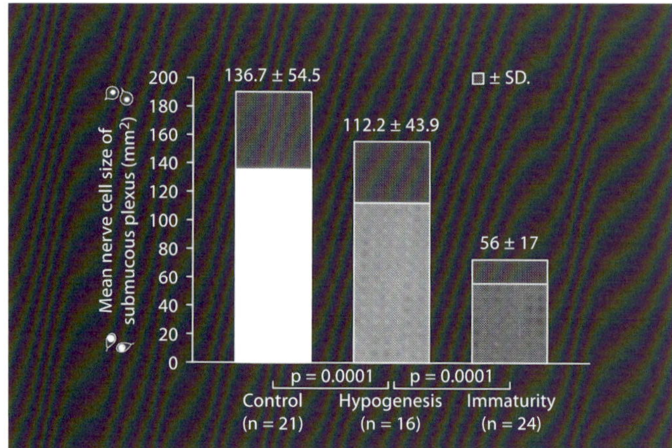

Fig. 42. Morphometric data demonstrating nerve cell size in normal, hypoganglionic, and immature submucous plexus.

Intestinal Neuronal Dysplasia Type A

Intestinal neuronal dysplasia type A (IND A) is a necrotizing enterocolitis (NEC; fig. 43, 44) caused by immaturity of the sympathetic nervous system in the distal colon. In normal babies, histochemical staining of sympathetic nerve fibers shows a dense net of sympathetic nerves which surround arterial vessels (fig. 45, 46) [124]. In IND A, the sympathetic nerves are more or less missing in mucosal biopsies with NEC. The moderate increase of AChE in parasympathetic nerve fibers was the reason to name this disease IND A. The absence of sympathetic synapses inside the ganglia of the myenteric plexus (fig. 47–50) and the reactive increased parasympathetic tonus is possibly the reason for focal spasms of the colon.

The fact that NEC is mainly a disease of premature babies makes it easy to understand that with a colostoma in the ascending colon, NEC heals up in the distal colon at an age of about 8 months – a time at which sympathetic innervation has normalized. Cases which are not cured by 10 months of age may possibly suffer from sympathetic aplasia in the gut.

Disturbed blood flow and decreased mucous production seem to be the main pathogenetic factors of NEC. However, leukocytic infiltration of the intestinal wall has serious consequences concerning gut peristalsis. Leukocytic collagenases digest the tendinous network of circular and longitudinal muscles which cause focal atrophic desmosis (see section on atrophic desmosis). Peristalsis ends where the tendinous structure of the intestinal tract disappears. Chronic constipation is a consequence of atrophic desmosis [108, 125].

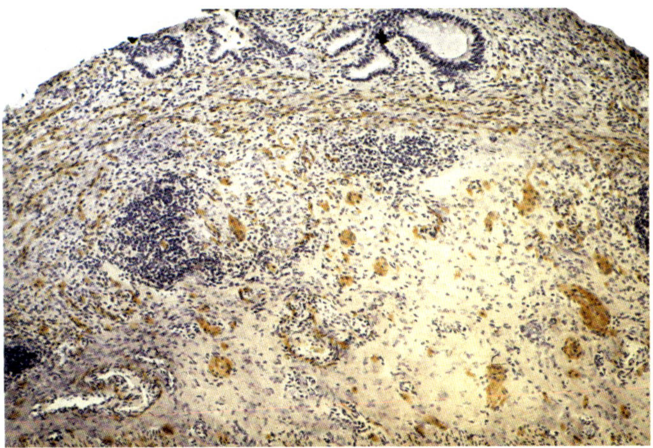

Fig. 43. NEC in IND A. AChE reaction with hemalum counterstaining. ×300.

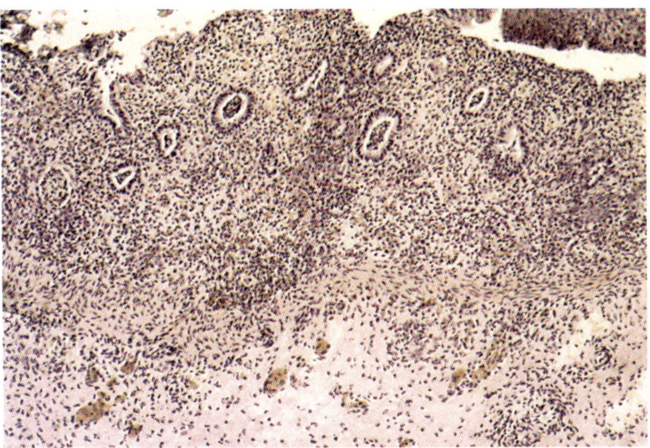

Fig. 44. Inflammation of colon mucosa in NEC (IND A) with microabscesses in tubular glands. AChE reaction with hemalum counterstaining. ×300.

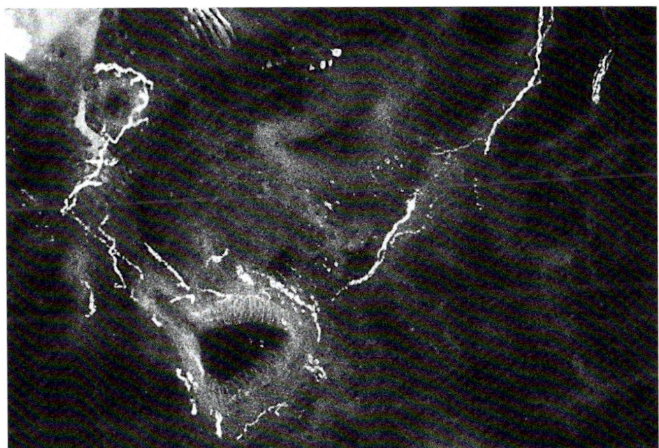

Fig. 45. Catecholamine-positive sympathetic nerves in the adventitia of submucous arterial vessels in normal colon. ×400.

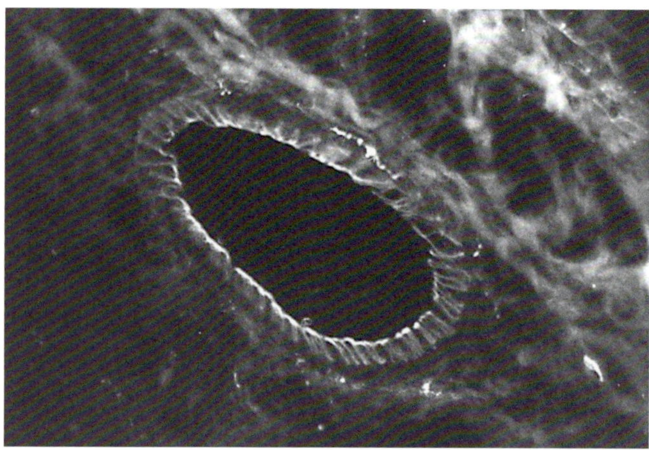

Fig. 46. No catecholaminergic nerves in the adventitia of arterial vessels in the submucosa of a biopsy with NEC (IND A; compare with fig. 45). Falck-Hillarp technique. ×480.

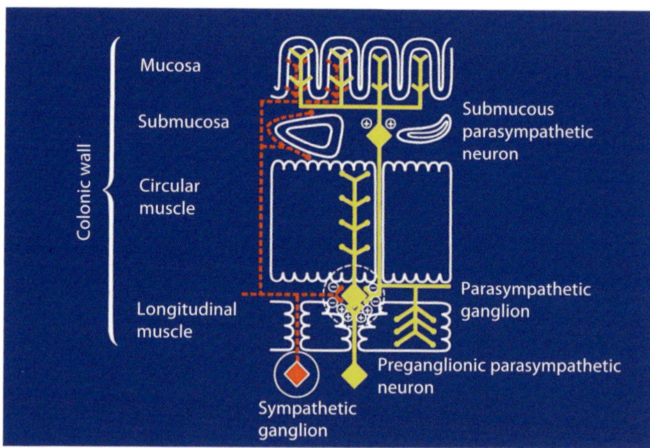

Fig. 49. Schematic drawing of normal sympathetic innervation (red lines).

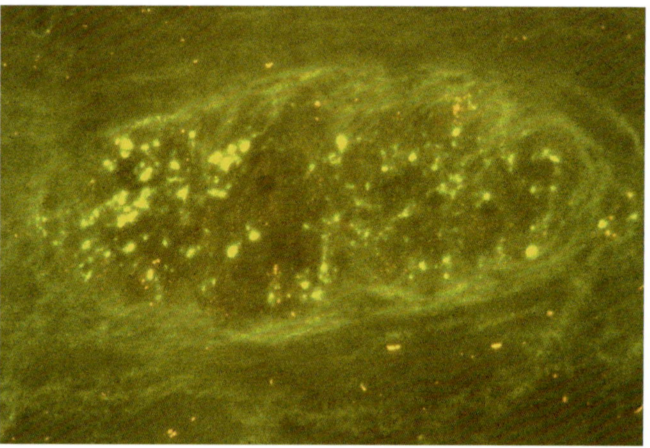

Fig. 47. Ganglion of the myenteric plexus with normal content of sympathetic synapses. Falck-Hillarp technique. ×600.

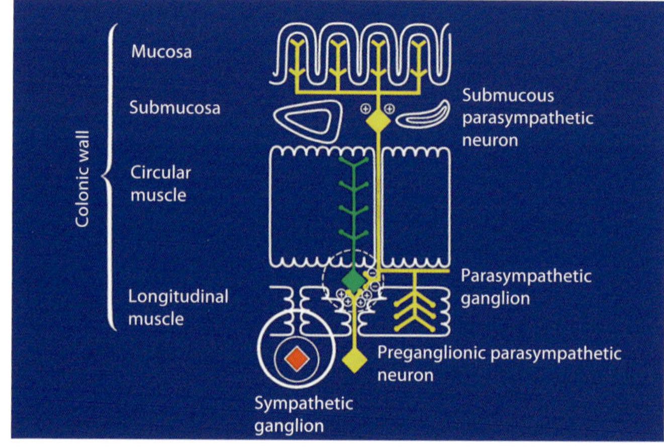

Fig. 50. Schematic representation of the lack of sympathetic innervation in the myenteric plexus, arterial vessels, and mucosa in IND A (NEC).

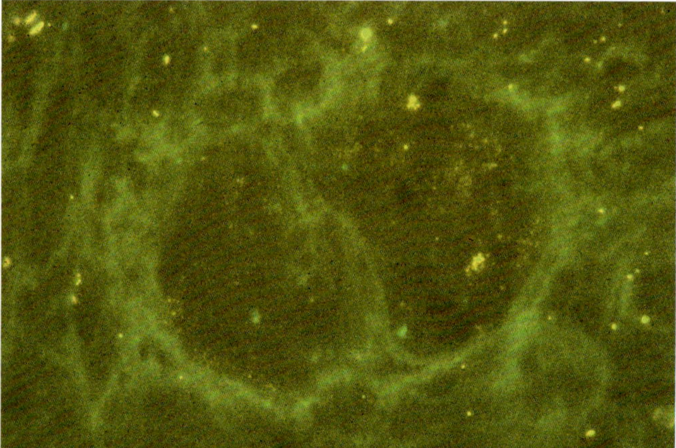

Fig. 48. Ganglion of the myenteric plexus without sympathetic synapses in IND A (compare with fig. 47). Falck-Hillarp technique. ×600.

Histopathology of Chronic Constipation

Intestinal Neuronal Dysplasia Type B

Since the first description of a case report of intestinal neuronal dysplasia type B (IND B) in 1971 [126], the diagnostic criteria have progressively improved along with the growing experience with the condition. We have learned that IND is not a qualitative diagnosis like HD, but rather a quantitative diagnosis [127]. Morphometric examinations of the plexus submucosus have shown that in 30 serial sections, about 20% of all ganglia must be giant ganglia with more than 8 nerve cells in IND B. This means that at least 4 giant ganglia (fig. 51) have to be registered in 30 serial sections.

A single giant ganglion has to be considered as an incidental finding [128]. A missing differentiation between nerve cells and glia cells must be interpreted as immaturity (fig. 52). Therefore, diagnosis of IND B should not be made before the first year of life [129, 130].

Diagnostic Criteria of Intestinal Neuronal Dysplasia Type B

1. IND B is an anomaly of the submucous plexus.
2. A reliable diagnosis needs about 16% giant ganglia, i.e. 4 to 5 giant ganglia in 30 serial sections.
3. Giant ganglia are global structures with more than 8 nerve cells in a ganglion cross-section. Normal submucous ganglia are disk-like structures (fig. 53).
4. Diagnosis of IND B should not be made before the first year of life.

IND B is frequently accompanied by immaturity of the enteric nervous system. This explains a normalization of colon motility in long-term clinical follow-up [120, 131, 132]. A morphometric quantification of the submucous plexus of healthy adult volunteers (n = 37) has shown no single case with IND B [133]. Conservative management is possible in most children with IND B [120, 134]. IND B has the capacity for functional normalization [135].

IND B is an anomaly of the submucous plexus; therefore, mucosal biopsies are sufficient for a diagnosis. However, with therapy-resistant constipation, hypoganglionosis of the myenteric plexus, desmosis, or an architectural malformation of the muscularis propria needs to be excluded [136].

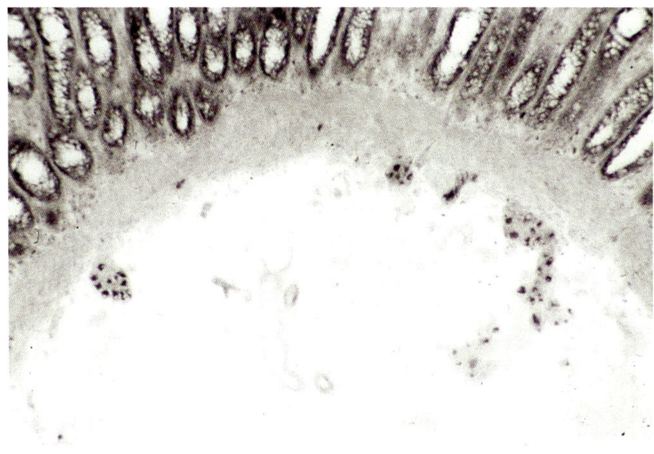

Fig. 51. IND B with two giant ganglia. LDH reaction. ×160.

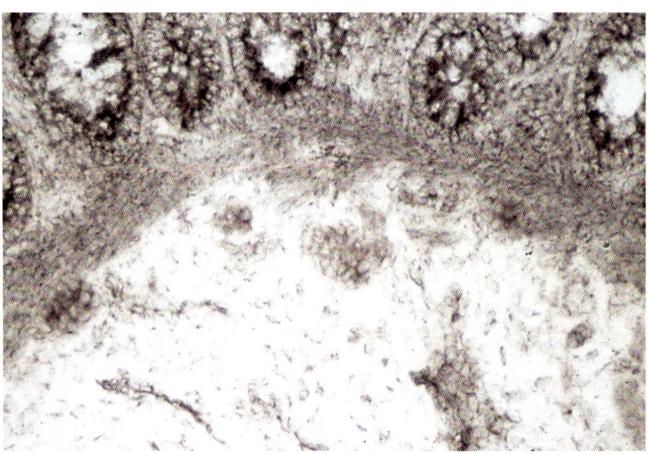

Fig. 52. Immature submucous plexus with pseudo-giant ganglia (4-month-old boy). ×180.

The combination of HD and IND B (proximal of an aganglionosis) supports the idea that IND B is a developmental anomaly (fig. 54) [38, 137–139]. No genetic defects could be demonstrated in man [137, 140, 141]; only in heterozygous endothelin B-deficient rats could characteristics of IND B with giant ganglia be observed [142, 143]. From a clinical point of view, electromanometric registered missing anorectal reflex is helpful in screening IND patients [144, 145].

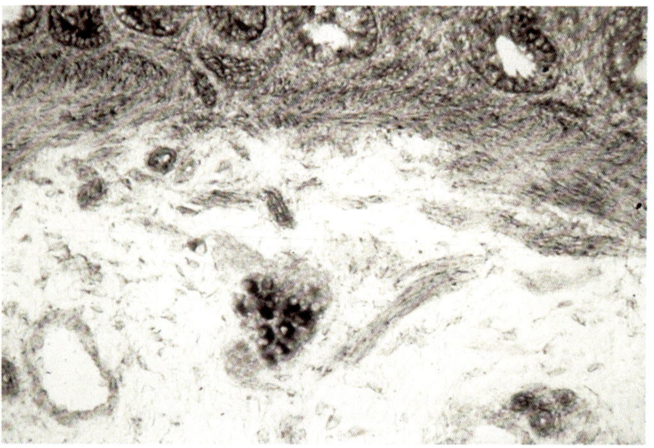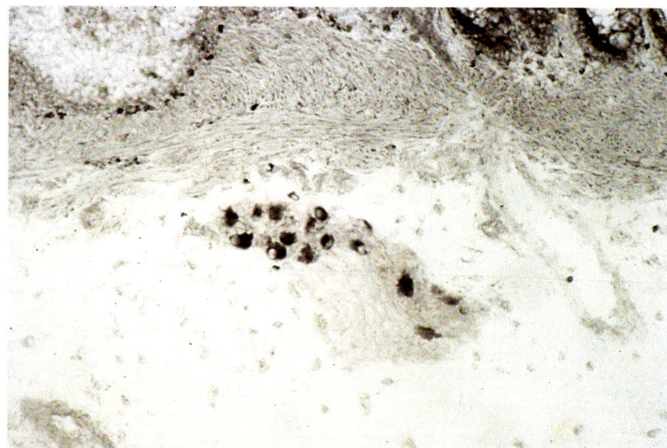

Fig. 53. Giant ganglia with more than 8 nerve cells. NOS reaction. ×180.

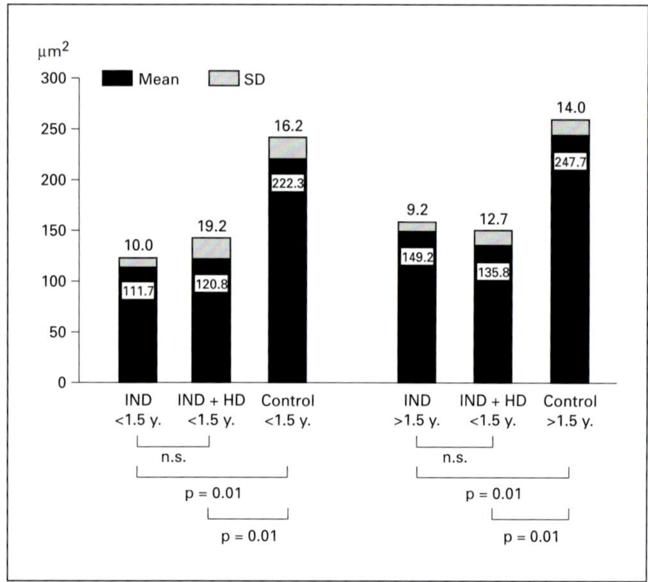

Fig. 54. Morphometric determinations of nerve cell sizes in the submucous plexus demonstrating significantly smaller nerve cells in IND B than in normal mucosa biopsies.

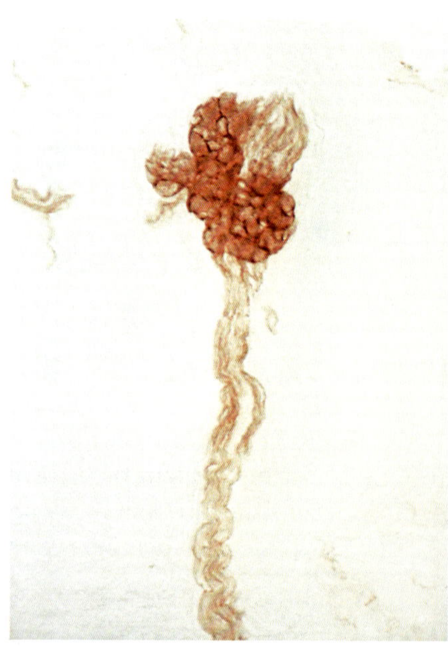

Fig. 55. Spherical giant ganglion surrounding an afferent submucous nerve fiber. AChE reaction. ×300.

Clinical Indications of Intestinal Neuronal Dysplasia Type B

1 Missing anorectal reflex.
2 IND B is often combined with distal aganglionosis or hypoganglionosis of the myenteric plexus.
3 Most cases with IND B and constipation normalize by 4 years of age with apoptosis of the submucous plexus.

The fact that IND shows giant ganglia along afferent parasympathetic nerves generates the impression that invasion of neuroblasts from the myenteric plexus is stopped during the distribution of ganglia and nerve cells in the submucous plexus (fig. 55) [2].

Unlike HD, diagnosis of IND does not need native tissue. It can be diagnosed in formalin-fixed and paraffin-embedded tissue by immunohistochemical techniques, i.e. PGP 9.5 [146], MAP 2 [147], and cathepsin D with osmium tetroxide contrast [148, 149].

IND B has also been diagnosed in adults with primary chronic constipation [150, 151]. In these cases the question was discussed if a prolonged intestinal obstruction may be responsible for initiating the development of giant ganglia. This, however, could not be proven [152].

B.10

Ganglioneuromatosis. Multiple Endocrine Neoplasia 2B (MEN 2B)

It is important to be aware that ganglioneuromatosis multiple endocrine neoplasia 2B (MEN 2B) causes Hirschsprung symptomatology. It is sometimes misdiagnosed as IND B. Giant ganglia in MEN 2B are much bigger than the giant ganglia of IND B (fig. 56, 57). In addition, nerve fiber proliferations with high AChE activity can be observed (fig. 58) [2, 153]. Early and reliable diagnosis of ganglioneuromatosis is important because many of these patients develop time-dependent MEN. MEN 2B is associated quite early with the development of a medullary thyroid carcinoma, a pheochromocytoma, or hyperparathyroidism. In the literature, many case reports describe ganglioneuromas, medullary thyroid carcinoma with high calcitonin plasma levels, and pheochromocytoma [154–157].

Glia cell line-derived neurotrophic factor and neurotrophic factor neuroturin play an important role in the pathogenesis of ganglioneuromatosis [158]. These factors are also expressed in the cells of a thyroid adenocarcinoma.

In native tissue, AChE and a LDH or NADH reaction allow a reliable diagnosis. The giant ganglia of ganglioneuromatosis contain 12–30 nerve cells. In paraffin sections, an immunohistochemical reaction of S 100, MAP 2, and osmium-enhanced cathepsin D may be helpful for making a diagnosis.

The excessive hyperplasia of the submucous plexus is the result of a high level of nerve growth factor.

HD and ganglioneuromatosis are considered to be a dominant inherited neurocristopathy due to RET gene mutations [155, 159]. This combination is obviously extremely rare. Case reports of MEN 2B and a short Hirschsprung have only been described in 2 patients [160].

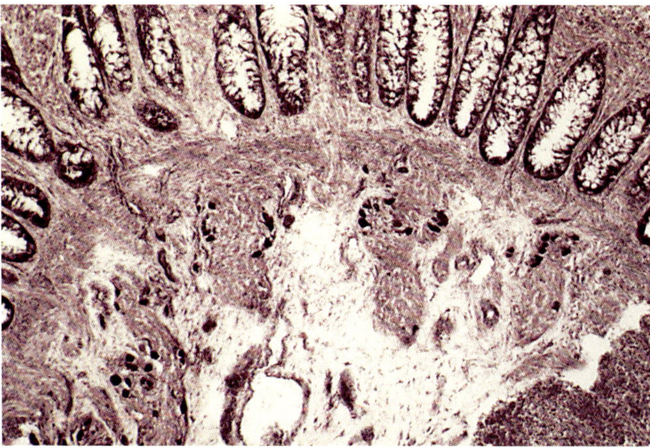

Fig. 56. Ganglioneuromatosis (MEN 2B) with many giant ganglia in a hyperplastic submucous plexus. LDH reaction. ×180.

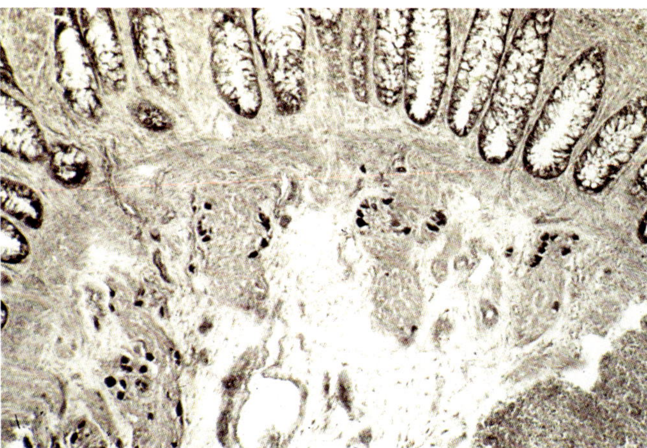

Fig. 57. MEN 2B with an accumulation of giant ganglia. NOS reaction. ×180.

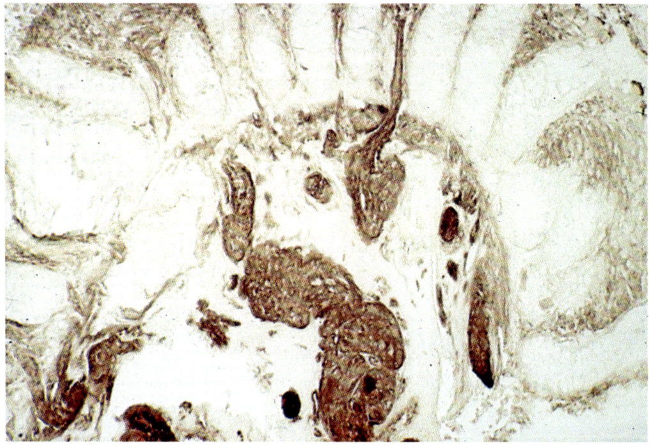

Fig. 58. Nerve fiber proliferation in MEN 2B with increased AChE activity. ×180.

A loss of tendinous structures in circular and longitudinal muscles and a loss of the myenteric tendinous plexus fascia are characteristic lesions in desmosis coli which abolish a directed peristalsis.

In order to understand the functional mechanisms of the tendinous structures in the intestinal wall, it is worthwhile to go several decades back to the anatomical investigation of Goertler [161]. Goertler demonstrated that peristalsis not only needs an enteric nervous system and smooth muscles of the muscularis propria, but also a tendinous net in circular and longitudinal muscles anchored in the connective tissue fascia of the myenteric plexus layer.

We know that circular and longitudinal muscles contract and relax alternatively. Through contraction, the tendinous network of circular muscles stretches relaxed longitudinal muscles, and the contraction of longitudinal muscles dilates relaxed circular muscles (fig. 59, 60). The tendinous networks of circular and longitudinal muscles are positioned at a 90° angle to each other. For the morphological inspection of both tendinous nets in the two muscle layers, it is necessary to cut the intestinal wall in a 45° angle, related to the length and transversal position of the gut. If the muscularis propria is cut in an exact longitudinal direction, only the plexus layer and the tendinous fiber net of circular muscles are seen. Exact transversal cutting of the gut only shows the plexus layer and tendinous net of longitudinal muscles.

Smooth muscles preserve connective tissue fibers of the intestinal wall. Picrosirius red staining proved to generate the highest contrast between collagen fibers and smooth muscles in cryostat or paraffin sections. Native tissue sections require Delaunay fixation before picrosirius red staining.

Aplastic Desmosis

Aplastic desmosis is a characteristic anomaly in the megacystis microcolon syndrome. It is accompanied by an intestinal pseudo-obstruction. This syndrome is considered to be an autosomal recessive disorder [162–166]. Histological examination of the muscularis propria in the jejunum, ileum, and colon shows a complete lack of tendon-like connective tissue net in circular and longitudinal muscles. No tendinous connective tissue layer be-

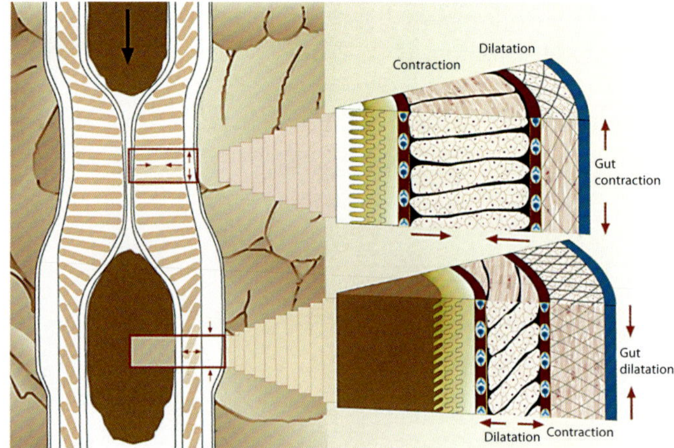

Fig. 59. Normal movement of muscularis propria. Schematic representation of stretching the gut wall by contraction of circular muscles by the tendinous network (top), while longitudinal muscles are relaxed. Dilatation of the gut is operated by contraction of longitudinal muscles and its tendinous net, fixed to the connective tissue layer between both muscle compartments (bottom). Both movements characterize peristalsis.

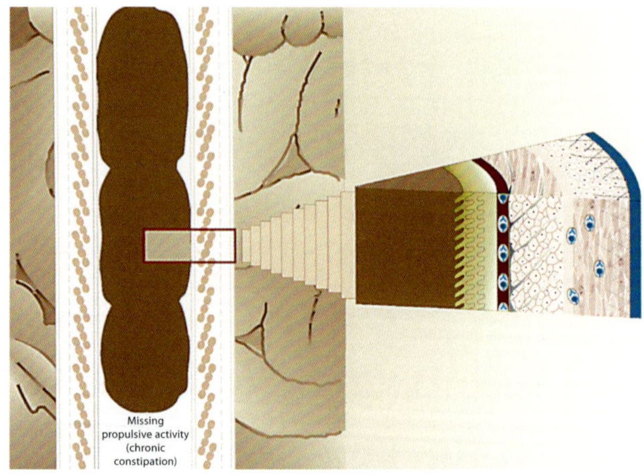

Fig. 60. Missing continuity of connective tissue net in the muscularis propria. Schematic drawing of the missing muscle mechanics in desmosis by a missing connective tissue plexus layer and the internal tendinous nets in circular and longitudinal muscles [219].

tween the circular and longitudinal muscles has been observed (fig. 61–64) [167–172].

Alterations in the smooth muscle cytoskeleton and contractile proteins are considered to be the reason of the megacystis microcolon syndrome with gut aperistalsis [173–175]. Other authors have observed an anti-smooth

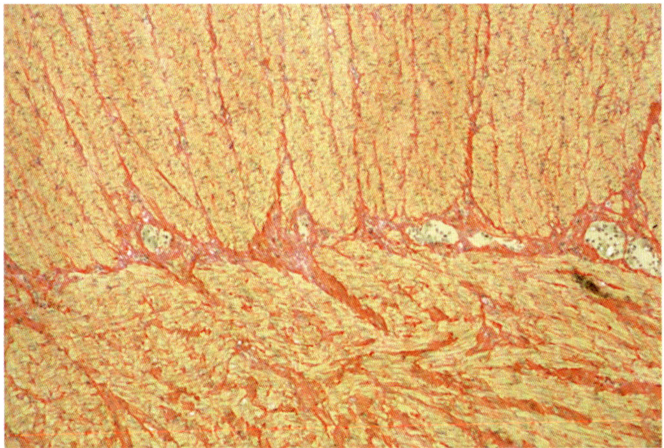

Fig. 61. Normal ascending colon with well-developed connective tissue plexus layer and tendinous fiber nets in longitudinal and circular muscles. Picrosirius red staining; 45° cutting angle. ×120.

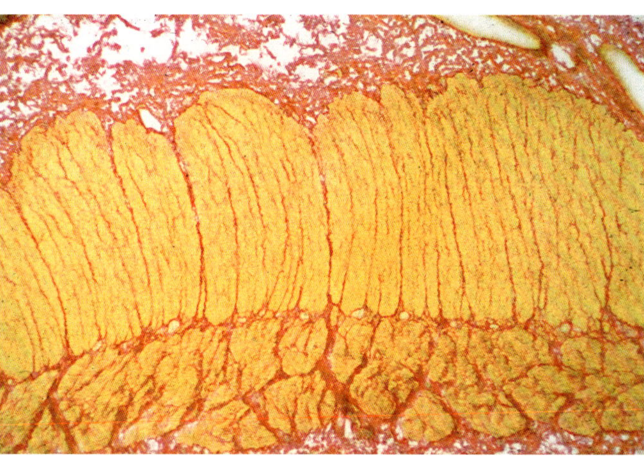

Fig. 63. Normal ileum with well-developed tendinous nets in ring and length muscles. Connective tissue layer between circular and longitudinal muscles. Picrosirius red staining; 45° cutting angle. ×80.

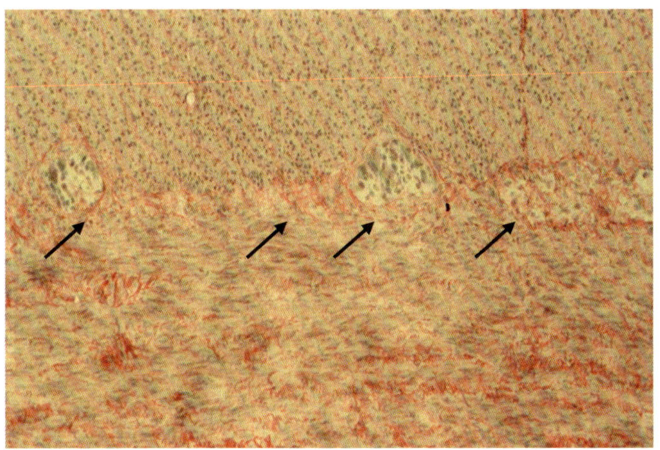

Fig. 62. Ascending colon with aplastic desmosis. Well-developed myenteric plexus (arrows) but missing connective tissue structures in muscularis propria (compare with fig. 61). Picrosirius red staining. ×120.

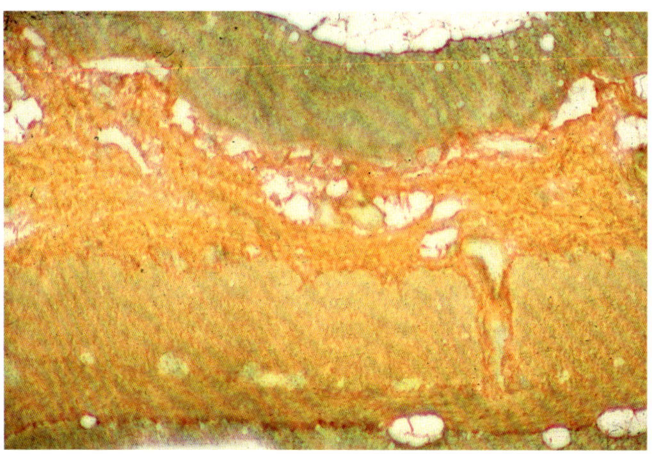

Fig. 64. Ileum with aplastic desmosis and atrophy of muscularis propria. Picrosirius red staining. ×80.

muscle protein [176]. Ultrastructural studies have demonstrated degenerative lesions of gut smooth muscles [177]. Diminished expression of enteric α-smooth-muscle actin has also been described [178].

Altogether, a defect of smooth muscle metabolism is responsible for the missing development of the tendinous structures in the muscularis propria. This lesion is characteristic for the megacystis microcolon syndrome, a defect which develops in the 9th to 10th embryonic week [19]. The disease seems to occur more frequently in females than males [168, 179].

A physiological aplasia of tendinous structures in the muscularis propria is always observed in the vermiform appendix (fig. 65). The increased AChE activity of the parasympathetic innervation of the appendix (fig. 66–68) also explains the missing peristalsis and permanent spasticity of the vermiform appendix.

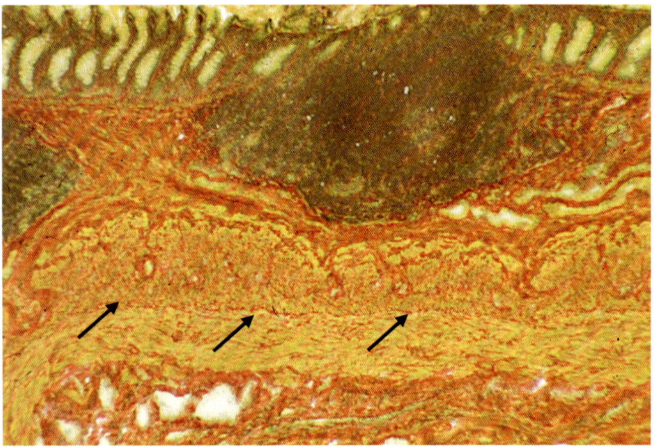

Fig. 65. Physiological aplasia of tendinous nets in muscularis propria of vermiform appendix. No connective tissue layer (arrows) between circular and longitudinal muscles. Picrosirius red staining. ×160.

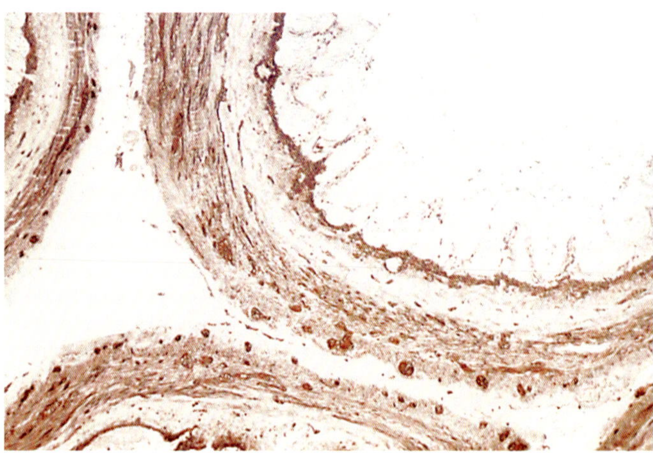

Fig. 67. Transverse section of vermiform appendix with typical high AChE activity in muscularis propria and mucosa. AChE reaction. ×16.

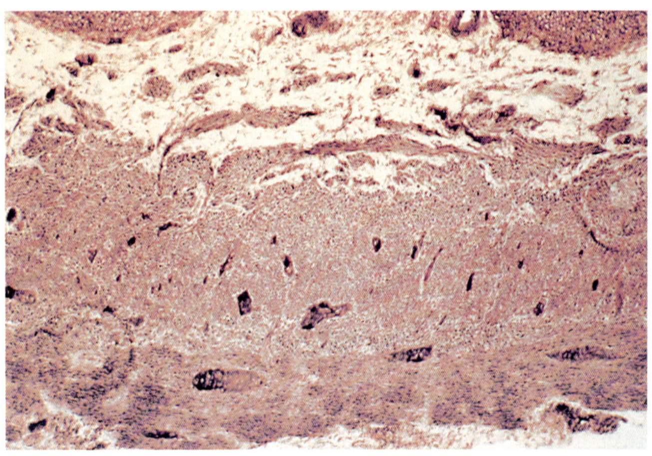

Fig. 66. Normal vermiform appendix with physiological heterotopic myenteric plexus in muscularis propria. LDH reaction. ×75.

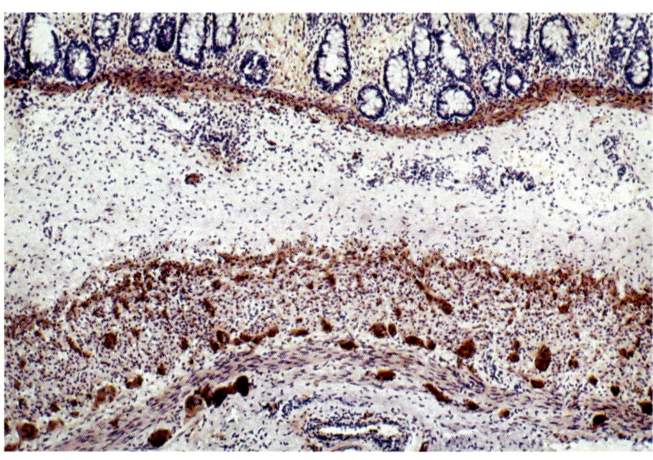

Fig. 68. Physiological increase of AChE in parasympathic nerve fibers and ganglia of muscularis mucosae and muscularis propria. This picture demonstrates permanent spasticity of vermiform appendix. AChE reaction with hemalum counterstaining. ×160.

Atrophic Desmosis

Inflammation of the muscularis propria, typical in Crohn's disease, NEC, and diverticulitis, is the reason for focal loss of tendinous net and plexus layer in muscularis propria. All of these lesions cause symptoms of a stenotic syndrome. In addition, postoperative X-ray irradiation of resected colon cancer causes a lesion in the muscularis propria with a focal loss of tendinous net of the plexus layer as well as circular muscles and longitudinal muscles. These patients develop stenotic symptoms, which from a clinical point of view are normally interpreted as cicatricial stenosis. Histological examination of these structures generally shows only an atrophy of the tendinous nets of circular and longitudinal muscles [180].

Focal atrophic desmosis in Crohn's disease (fig. 69, 70) and diverticulitis is caused by collagenases of inflammatory leukocytes which digest the tendinous collagen

Histopathology of Chronic Constipation

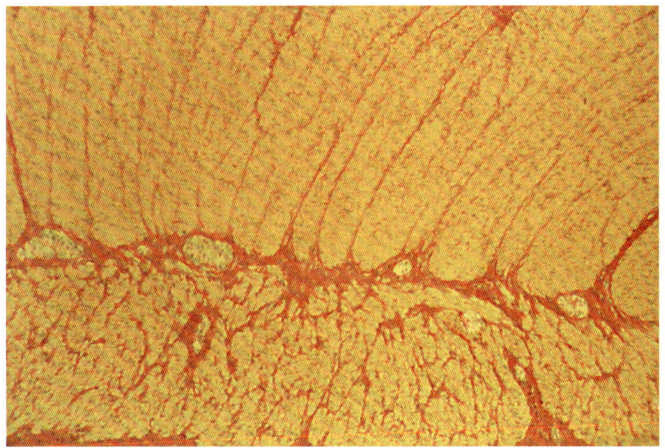

Fig. 69. Normal transverse colon section. Pricrosirius red staining; cutting angle 45°. ×180.

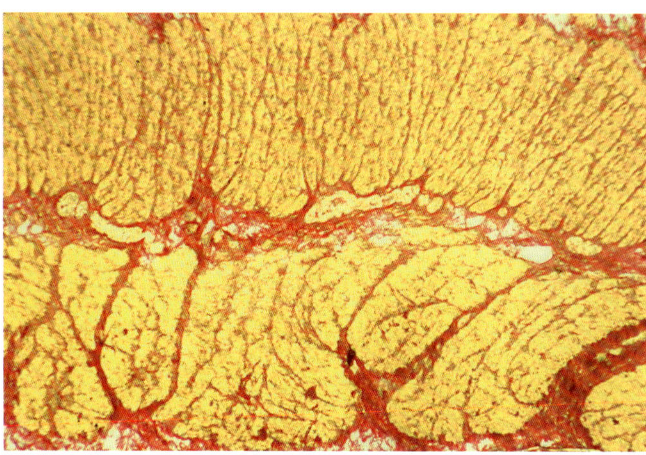

Fig. 71. Normal connective tissue structures in muscularis propria (staining and cutting angle as fig. 69).

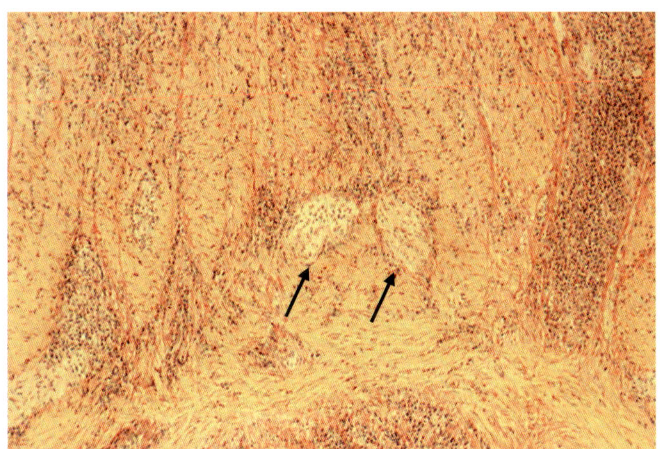

Fig. 70. Transverse colon with acute Crohn's disease and destruction of all collagen structures by leukocytic collagenases. Arrows show the myenteric plexus. Picrosirius red staining. ×180.

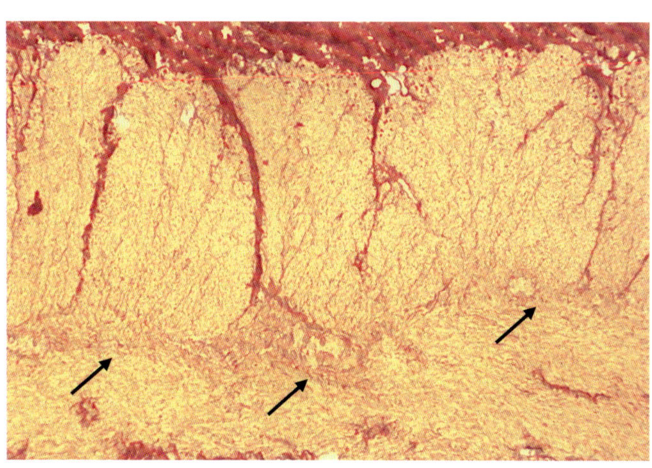

Fig. 72. Atrophic desmosis with loss of connective tissue plexus layer (arrows). Rests of the loop net of the connective tissue of the circular muscles can be observed. Picrosirius red staining; cutting angle 45°. ×74.

structures in the muscularis propria and plexus layer [169]. Peristalsis ends at that position in which tendinous connective tissue of the colonic wall has disappeared.

In colon with long-lasting chronic constipation the tendinous collagen structures atrophy intertaenially (fig. 71, 72). Only in the taeniae is the tendinous net of circular and longitudinal muscles, including the plexus layer, preserved (fig. 73). The resulting slow-transit constipation is obviously operated by taeniae, which show hypertrophy of the muscularis propria. These forms of desmosis coli are considered as 'incomplete desmosis'. Incomplete atrophic desmosis seems to be the result of an ischemic lesion in the muscularis propria by chronic constipation. Incomplete atrophic desmosis is often accompanied by focal atrophic alteration of longitudinal or circular muscles (fig. 73, 74) [181]. Even idiopathic megacolon is characterized by a complete loss of the tendinous net in muscularis propria [182].

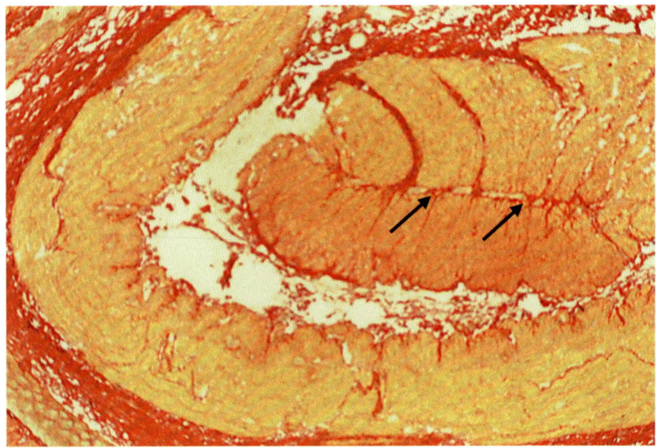

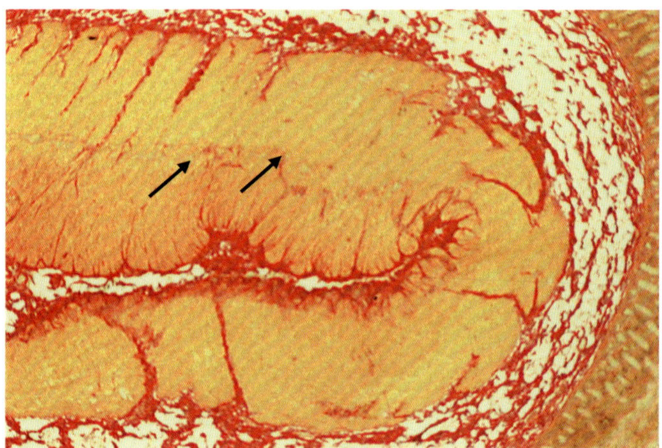

Fig. 73. Incomplete atrophic desmosis with a resting connective tissue plexus layer in the taeniae (arrows). Picrosirius red staining. ×48.

Fig. 74. Complete desmosis with atrophy of the connective tissue plexus layer (arrows; compare with fig. 73). ×48.

Pathogenesis of Focal Atrophic Desmosis

1 NEC
2 Crohn's disease
3 Diverticulitis
4 Focal X-ray irradiation
5 Colitis
6 Stretching lesion of muscularis propria (incomplete desmosis)

B.12

Architectural Malformation of the Muscularis Propria

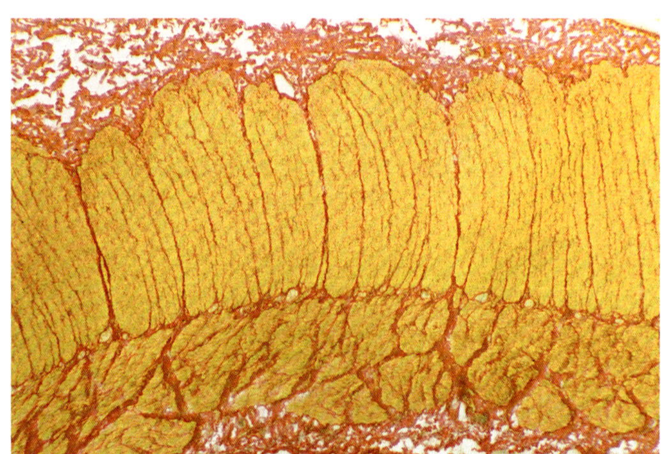

Fig. 75. Normal tendinous nets of circular and longitudinal muscles. Well-developed connective tissue plexus layer. Picrosirius red staining; cutting angle 45°. ×180.

The development of two myenteric plexus layers is accompanied by a serious pseudo-obstruction [136, 183]. This anomaly demonstrates that peristalsis of the gut, which is operated by an alternative contraction or relaxation of circular and longitudinal muscles, is blocked if this gut movement is not possible. The malformation of a doubling of the myenteric plexus layer (fig. 75–78) does not allow a coordinated movement of circular and longitudinal muscles (fig. 59, 60).

If this anomaly is a localized lesion of the colon or ileum, it can be effectively treated by surgical means. If architectural malformations concern the complete gut, an aperistaltic syndrome results and gut transplantation may be considered [136]. Recent genetic studies have shown that abnormal layering of the muscularis propria is a seldom-observed disease, but does seem to be a hereditary disorder [183].

A doubling of the myenteric plexus layer is normally accompanied by a hypoplastic hypoganglionosis (fig. 76). A normal construction of the tendinous net in longitudinal and circular muscles is missing; therefore, no coordinated peristalsis is possible (fig. 73, 74). Bioptic verification of this disease is possible from seromuscular biopsies taken laparoscopically.

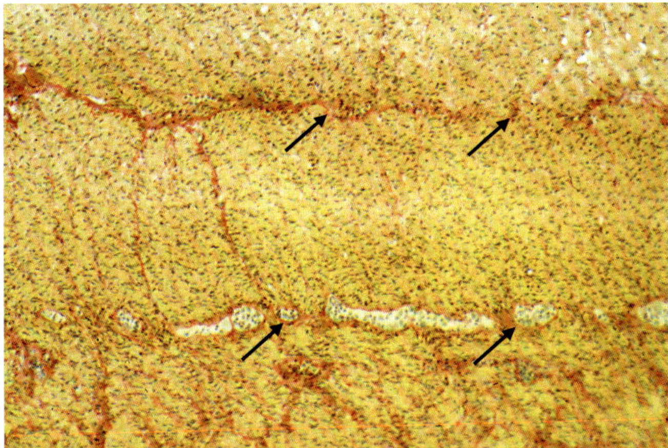

Fig. 76. Doubling of myenteric plexus layer (arrows) and abnormal tendinous net in muscularis propria (compare with fig. 75) ×180.

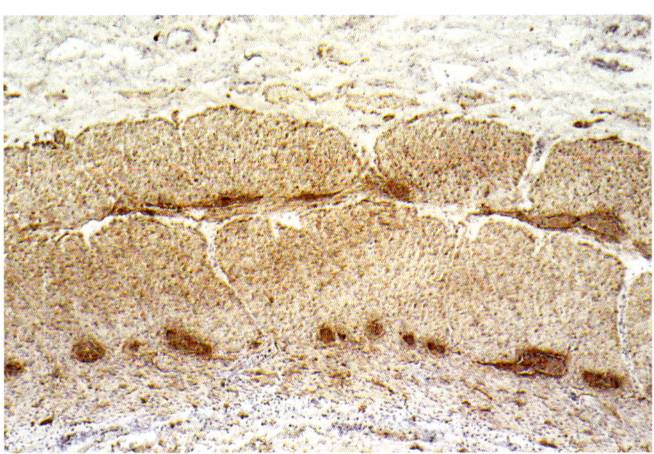

Fig. 77. Doubling of myenteric plexus. AChE reaction. ×120.

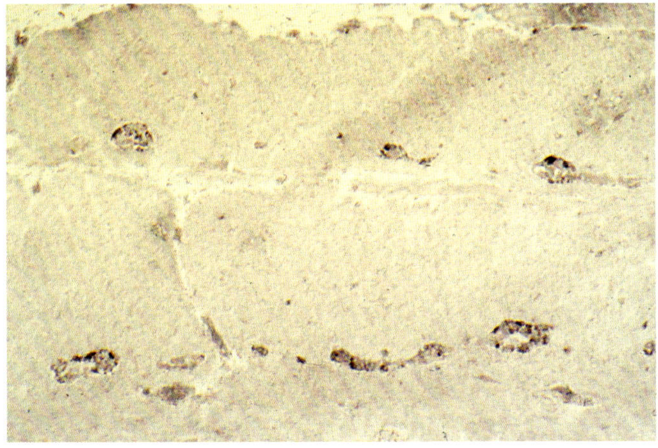

Fig. 78. Doubling of myenteric plexus. LDH reaction. ×120.

Degenerative Leiomyopathy: A Rare Disease

Based on current knowledge, pseudo-obstruction due to leiomyopathy is rare in the Western world. Only in the African population is a familiar degenerative hollow visceral myopathy described [184–189]. In contrast to the African population, in Caucasians a hereditary visceral myopathy is mainly observed in adults. All described cases were postulated to be an autoimmune disease [190, 191]. In most case reports describing familial visceral myopathy, however, it is not mentioned if the patients described are African or not [192–194].

Visceral muscular disorder may arise in the context of muscular dystrophy, progressive systemic sclerosis, Ehlers-Danlos syndrome or collagenosis-like systemic lupus erythematosus, dermatomyositis, or primary visceral myopathy [195].

The so-called hollow visceral myopathies, which are observed in African people, affect the gastrointestinal tract, descending urinary tract, and gallbladder [195]. These myopathies constitute the most common causes of primary chronic intestinal pseudo-obstruction, with a female predominance. The familial myopathies with variable modes of transmission are separated from sporadic forms [196, 197]. A relation to glycogenosis type IV or polysaccharidosis has been described [198, 199].

The clinical manifestation shows a broad spectrum with initial symptoms in the second decade up to middle age, ranking from dysphagia to alternating constipation, diarrhea, and volvulus. Microscopically, all muscular layers of the intestinal tract may be involved as well as the vascular walls. The muscle cells show cytoplasmic clearing, inclusions, rarefication, and vacuolation with caliber variation (fig. 79, 80) [198, 200].

Visceral myopathies may be a manifestation of a mitochondriopathy with various neuromuscular abnormalities [201]. One of the most important entities is the autosomal recessive mitochondrial neurogastrointestinal encephalomyopathy. Mitochondrial myopathies are characterized by an association of gastrointestinal, neuromuscular, and nonneuromuscular symptoms with maternal inheritance [195].

Over a period of 50 years, only two European adults with visceral myopathy were observed at the Basel Institute of Pathology. These patients showed atrophy of smooth muscle fibers with inclusion bodies in muscle fibers of the colon (fig. 81, 82) and a loss of immunohistochemical ex-

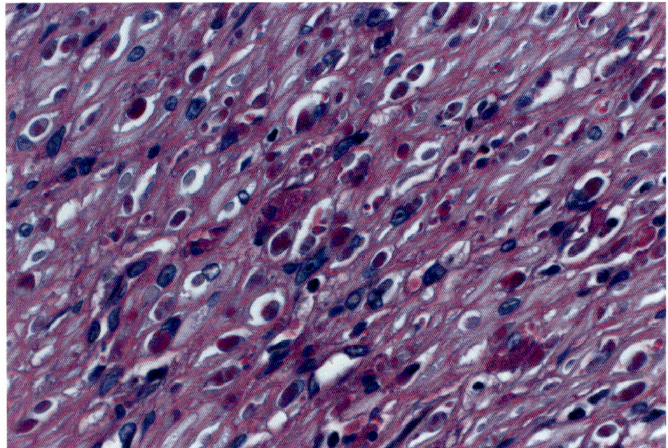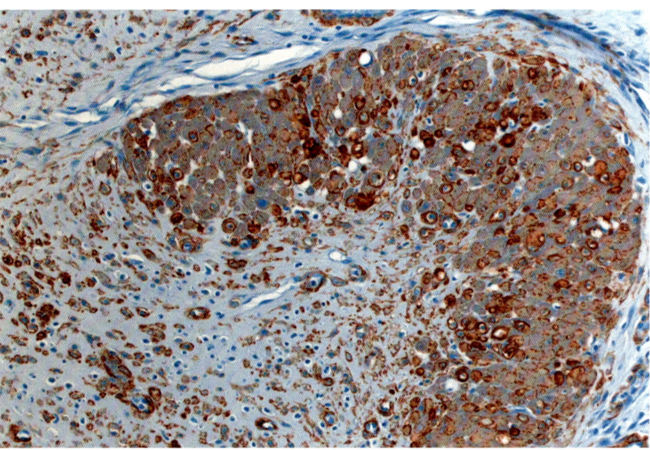

Fig. 79. Leiomyopathy with atrophy of tendinous tissue nets in circular (arrow) and longitudinal muscles (double arrows). Atrophy of connective tissue plexus layer. Picrosirius red staining. ×120.

Fig. 80. Colon wall with normal tendinous connective tissue net in circular and longitudinal muscles. Well-developed connective tissue plexus layer. Picrosirius red staining. ×90.

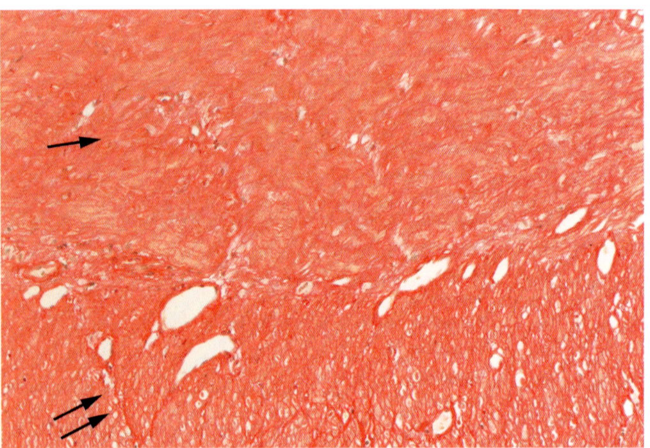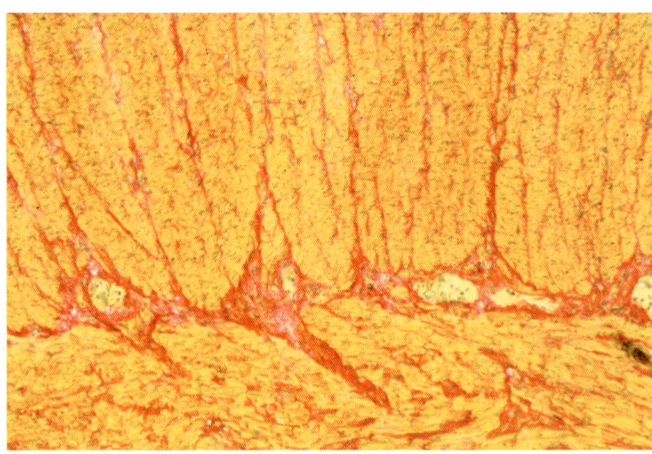

Fig. 81. Leiomyopathy with PAS-positive inclusion bodies (arrow) in the circular muscles of the colon wall. ×200.

Fig. 82. Degenerative leiomyopathy with loss of immunohistochemical vimentin-stained smooth muscles of colon. ×80.

pression of vimentin and actin (fig. 82). Atrophy of smooth muscles was accompanied by atrophy of the tendinous nets in circular and longitudinal muscles (fig. 79, 80). No signs of inflammation were observed. Both patients died from the myopathy and the intestinal obstruction.

Schuffler and Beegle [196] differentiated degenerative visceral myopathy and hereditary hollow visceral myopathy as two different diseases of intestinal smooth muscles.

Myopathies are interpreted as a mesenchymopathy [202, 203]. In a few papers, a genetic etiology of visceral myopathy in Europeans is postulated [204, 205].

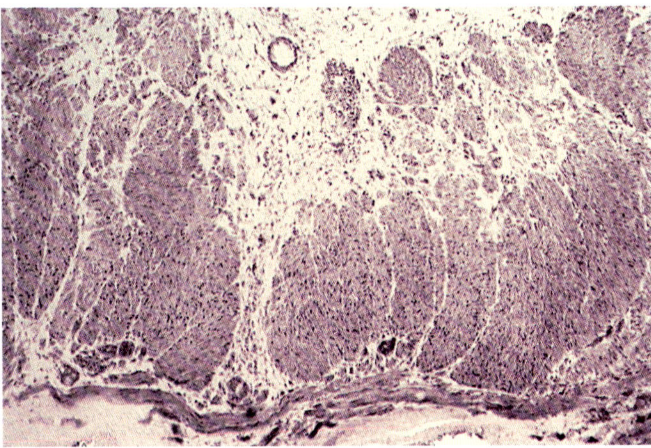

Fig. 83. Ascending colon with severe distension atrophy of circular and longitudinal muscles caused by an atrophic desmosis. LDH reaction. ×120.

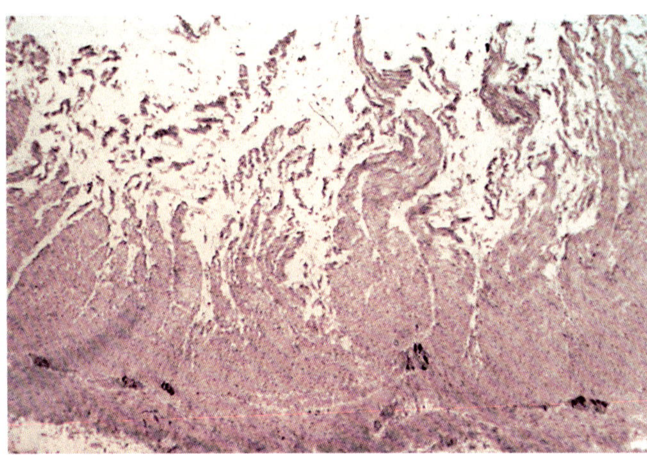

Fig. 84. Distention atrophy of circular muscles of proximal ascending colon caused by chronic constipation due to a hypoplastic hypoganglionosis. LDH reaction. ×120.

B.14

Stretching Atrophy of Circular and Longitudinal Muscles in the Gut

Focal stretching atrophy of the inner layer of circular muscles can be frequently observed in adults, but sometimes also in chronically constipated children. Two different forms have been observed: atrophy of the inner layer of circular muscles (fig. 83, 84) and atrophy of circular muscles below the dehydrogenase-rich last inner layer of circular muscles (fig. 83–86).

These lesions are mainly seen in the distal colon and are accompanied by an increase of connective scar tissue in the atrophic muscles. They are mainly observed in dehydrogenase reactions and are sometimes hard to be objectified in HE staining. A scar can be demonstrated quite clearly in a picrosirius red staining [206]. Shrinkage phenomena by formalin fixation frequently mask stretching artefacts in circular muscles.

In a few cases, focal scars have been observed in longitudinal muscles (fig. 85). Scars and muscle atrophy in the muscularis propria are accompanied by chronic constipation because alternative stretching and contraction of longitudinal and circular muscles are no longer possible. Disturbed peristalsis is the consequence of this alteration.

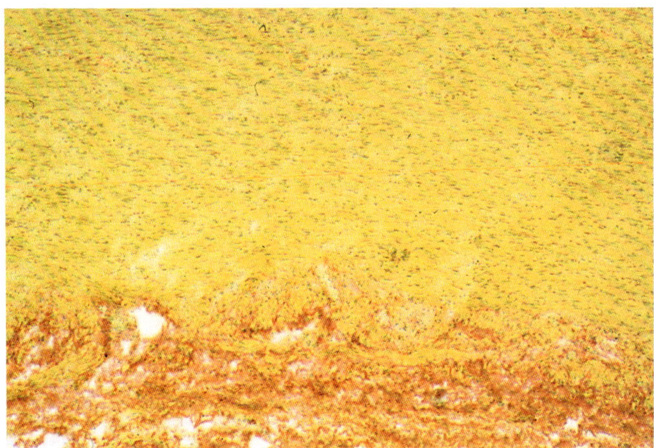

Fig. 85. Atrophic longitudinal muscles with scar tissue. Atrophy of tendinous net in muscularis propria and plexus layer. Picrosirius red staining. ×120.

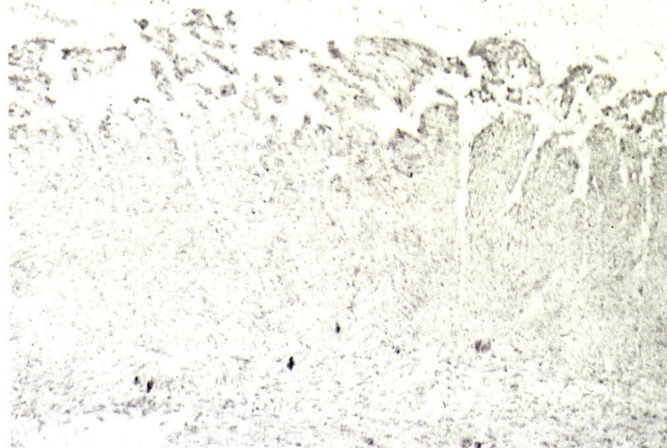

Fig. 86. Distension atrophy of circular muscles due to atrophic hypoganglionosis. LDH reaction. ×120.

Nerve Cell Heterotopias in Mucosa and Muscularis Propria

It is important to distinguish nerve cell heterotopias in colon mucosa from nerve cell heterotopias of the myenteric plexus in longitudinal muscles.

The submucous plexus often shows nerve cells or ganglia in the longitudinal layer of muscularis mucosae. This is a consequence of a hypertrophy of muscularis mucosae. This phenomenon has no influence on colon motility and is only a passive embedding of ganglia or nerve cells of the submucous plexus in the increased thickness of the longitudinal layers of muscularis mucosae (fig. 87). It is an indirect indication that muscularis mucosae have developed a hypertrophy due to chronic constipation.

Additionally, heterotopic nerve cells in lamina propria mucosae are episodic findings. The translocation of nerve cells of the submucous plexus into lamina propria mucosae are caused by lymph nodes which develop in submucosa and invade in a secondary step into mucosa (fig. 87–89). It is a lymph node-induced dislocation of nerve cells of the submucous plexus into lamina propria mucosae that has no influence on colon motility [207].

Heterotopic ganglia of the myenteric plexus into longitudinal or circular muscles of muscularis propria are frequently caused by a loss of the connective tissue fascia of myenteric plexus. It is a normal finding in the vermiform appendix [208], mainly in circular muscles. Atrophic desmosis of the colon shows nerve cell and ganglia heterotopias in the longitudinal muscle layer of the muscularis propria. This phenomenon is an indication of disturbed colon motility due to atrophy of the tendinous nets in muscularis propria and the plexus layer (fig. 90, 91).

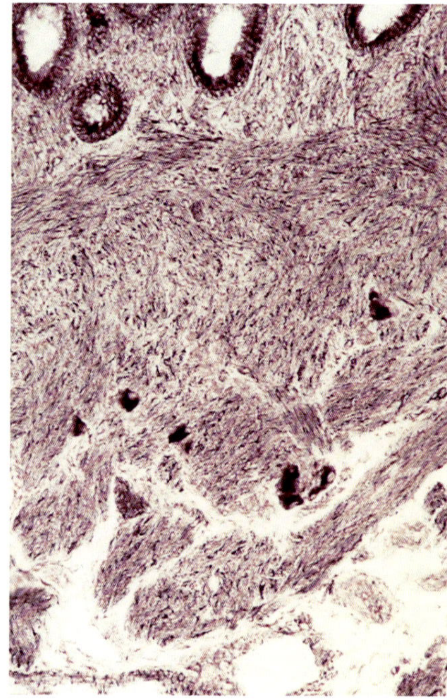

Fig. 87. Wrapping of submucous plexus by hypertrophic longitudinal muscles of muscularis mucosae. LDH reaction. ×120.

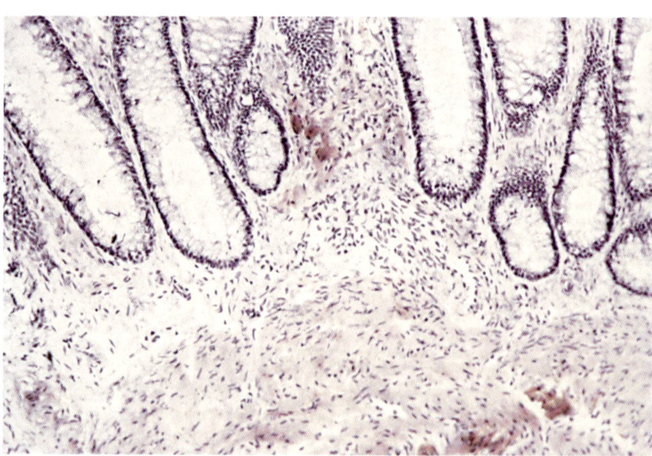

Fig. 88. Heterotopic nerve cells in lamina propria mucosae. AChE reaction with hemalum counterstaining. ×120.

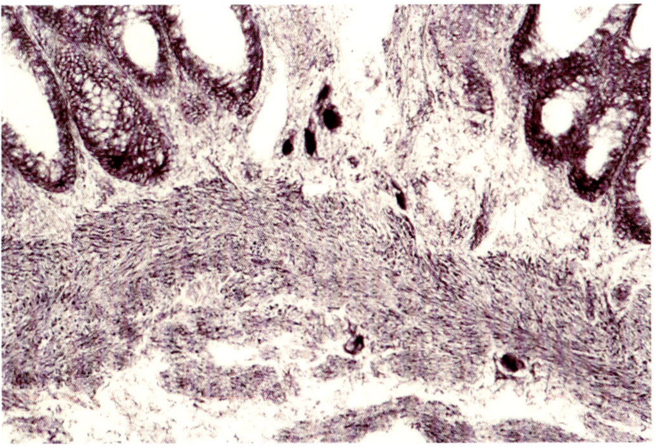

Fig. 89. Lymph node-induced dislocation of submucous nerve cells into lamina propria mucosae. LDH reaction. ×120.

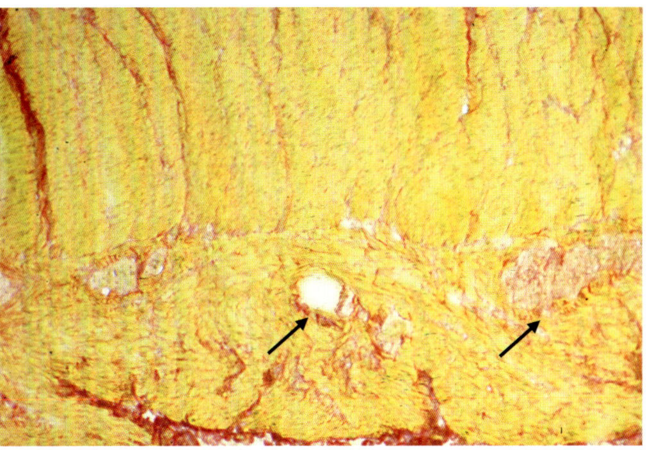

Fig. 91. Atrophic desmosis with heterotopic myenteric plexus (arrows) in longitudinal muscles. Picrosirius red staining. ×120.

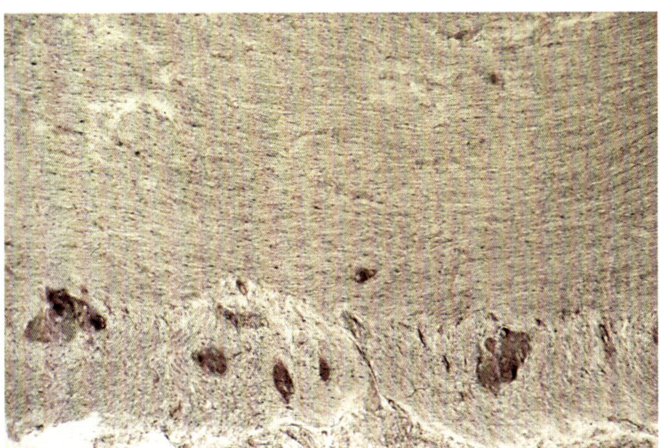

Fig. 90. Heterotopic myenteric plexus in longitudinal muscles due to an atrophic desmosis. LDH reaction. ×120.

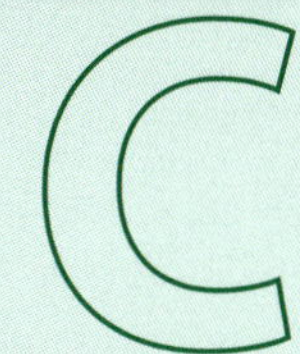

A Laboratory Guide to Histopathological Diagnosis of Intestinal Motility Disorders

Taking native rectum mucosa biopsies for a histopathological examination of chronic constipation has proven to be a simple and safe procedure, and may be the first diagnostic step in the diagnosis of chronic constipation [24].

For a functional disease like constipation, enzyme histochemistry is the technique of choice to evaluate an alteration of colon motility. In general terms, peristalsis depends on cholinergic innervation and sympathetic modulation in the myenteric plexus. An AChE reaction enables the pathologist to evaluate the actual gut tonus [32, 65, 152]. Decreased AChE activity in the colonic wall is a clear indication of disturbed motility, e.g. in hypoganglionosis of the myenteric plexus [106, 107]. In a similar way, nerve cell dehydrogenase activity (SDH) reflects nerve cell function, which is important in the evaluation of nerve cell immaturity of the enteric nervous system [22, 121].

The following section will demonstrate handling of native gut biopsies and the most important enzyme histochemical reactions in the daily pathohistological diagnostic routine in coloproctology and pediatric surgery.

C.1

The Most Important Technical Factors for Optimal Pathohistological Results

1 Enzyme histochemistry works with native tissue.
2 CO_2 frozen biopsies or surgical specimens are briefly thawed and assembled exactly rectangular to the mucosa surface on a cryostat carrier. Tissue is then immediately refrozen on CO_2 ($-80\,^\circ$C). A magnifying head lens may be helpful for orientation of seromuscular biopsies or whole-mount biopsies.
3 Thickness of cryostat sections may be 15 μm. End-thickness of the spread and dried cryostat section on a microscopic slide is about 4 μm.
4   Sections evaluated with reference to their enzyme activity are not counterstained.
5 Resected gut specimens must be cut open and washed under tap water. Fat tissue must be removed. A 1- to 2-cm wide and 15-cm long stripe is prepared and caudocranially wound up (Swiss-roll technique; fig. 12). The rolled specimen is again frozen on CO_2 ($-80\,^\circ$C). Afterwards, the specimen can be stored at $-24\,^\circ$C.
6 Cryostat sections are dried on microscopic slides at room temperature. Avoid freezing cryostat sections inside the cryostat as ice crystal formation may damage the section. Air-dried sections can be stored for

several days in a refrigerator (4°C) before the enzyme histochemical reactions are started.

7 Slide boxes may be used for storage of cryostat sections in a refrigerator. Sections may be warmed up in the slide box to room temperature (about 15 min) before incubation for different enzyme reactions. Use of a slide box helps avoid having condensed water on slides. The risk of storage of slides at –80°C is the development of ice crystals.

8 After enzyme histochemical reactions, a 15-min 4% formalin fixation is necessary. Shorter fixation periods carry the risk of gas bubbles developing above the enzyme-rich nerve cells (e.g. AChE-containing ganglia) or tissue structures.

9 Cryostat sections, stained for histological orientation with hemalum, must be coated with Crystal Mount® (Biomeda, Foster City, Calif., USA) to avoid a time-dependent fading of hemalum staining. Hemalum staining is best if the cryostat section is degreased in increasing alcohol concentrations.

10 To avoid reaction differences from one reaction to the other, it is recommended to prepare stock media of 1,000 or 2,000 ml, according to the expected number of incubations in a 6- to 9-month period. Medium may be bottled in sealed plastic bottles containing approximately 30 ml of medium, which is a sufficient amount for the incubation of 15 slides in a Hellendahl vessel. Sealed plastic bottles are stored in a refrigerator at –20 to –30°C.

11 Before use, frozen medium is thawed in hot tap water and warmed to the required incubation temperature of 37°C.

C.2

Recommendations for Taking Mucosal Biopsies in Chronic Constipation

A disadvantage of enzyme histochemistry is the fact that native tissue is indispensable. This causes problems if an experienced pathologist is not in the same place. This problem can be overcome by freezing biopsies with CO_2 (–80°C) or petrol ether stored in a –25°C refrigerator. Biopsies can be sent to the pathologist in a Styropor box with CO_2 pellets (2–5 kg) by express service. Mucosal biopsies should measure approximately 3–5 mm^3 (the size of a peppercorn) and must include a sufficient quantity of submucosa. For an enzyme histochemical differ-

ential diagnosis, the following positions for taking biopsies are recommended:

Hirschsprung's Disease

1 1 cm proximal dentate line
2 3–4 cm proximal dentate line
3 6–8 cm dentate line

Ultrashort Hirschsprung's Disease

1 Rectoanal transition zone to evaluate musculus corrugator cutis ani
2 1 cm proximal dentate line
3 3–4 cm proximal dentate line
4 6–8 cm proximal dentate line to exclude total colon aganglionosis or long-segment Hirschsprung

Intestinal Neuronal Dysplasia of Submucous Plexus

1 4 cm proximal dentate line
2 8 cm proximal dentate line
3 10 cm proximal dentate line

Biopsies need a sufficient amount of submucosa to evaluate anomaly of submucous plexus.

Immaturity or Hypogenesis of Submucous Plexus

1 2 cm proximal dentate line
2 4 cm proximal dentate line
3 6–8 cm proximal dentate line

Suspected Hypoganglionosis of Myenteric Plexus

Hypoganglionosis of the myenteric plexus cannot be proven in mucosa biopsies. It can only be suspected if low AChE is observed. Proof of hypoganglionosis requires laparoscopic seromuscular biopsies from sigmoid, descending, transversal, and ascending colon. No mucosa may be biopsied.

Instructions for Transportation of Colorectal Biopsies or Surgical Specimens

For transportation of frozen biopsies over long distances, the following procedure has proven useful:

1 Carefully place each biopsy on the wall of a nylon or polyethylene tube with a volume of approximately 5 ml. An Eppendorf tube is optimal. Do not manipulate the tissue in any way (wrap, press, etc.). Insert a plug to avoid evaporation of the tissue.
2 Clearly mark the tube with the patient's name and the distance of the biopsy from the anal ring. Use a water-resistant marker. Do not use self-adhesive labels as they tend to become detached at $-80°C$.
3 Freeze tube directly on dry ice (CO_2) at $-80°C$ or iso-pentane (or petrol ether) stored in a $-80°C$ refrigerator. Do not use liquid nitrogen, as this may cause the biopsy to crack. Shock-frozen tissue can be stored at $-25°C$.
4 Do not freeze biopsies in an ordinary freezer ($-25°C$) as ice crystals destroy the tissue.
5 Do not freeze biopsies in physiological saline solution.
6 Place frozen tube in an envelope or a plastic bag and store on dry ice. Do not put any dry ice in the envelope or tube.
7 Ensure that biopsies are not stored at $-25°C$ for longer than 2 weeks (risk of desiccation).
8 Pack the plastic bag with the biopsy tubes in a polystyrene box large enough to hold 3–5 kg of dry ice.
9 Enclose a note with the patient's name, date of birth, and symptoms. Also include the name and address of the sender.
10 For shipping over long distances, calculate that about 2 kg of CO_2 will evaporate in 24 h.

Preparation of Cryostat Sections from Biopsies and Colorectal Specimens

D.1

The Problem of Section Thickness

To be compatible to a 4-μm thick paraffin section, it is recommended to cut cryostat sections with a thickness of 15 μm. A cryostat section which is thawed, spread, and dried on a microscopic slide loses about 70% of its thickness (fig. 92–95). Therefore, the end-thickness of the slide is 4 $\pm$ 0.5 μm. This can be clearly demonstrated in a scanning electron microscope picture or a physical measuring device (fig. 96). The thickness of the cryostat section is important because the amount of tissue influences the enzyme reaction. A 4-μm cryostat section has an end-thickness of 1 $\pm$ 0.2 μm, which is hard to cut and often gives no satisfactory enzyme reaction because the amount of enzyme is below the enzymatic starting reaction. A comparison of enzyme reactions of different section thicknesses demonstrated that the thickness of the cryostat section may not be less than 8 μm.

If the enzyme reaction cannot be performed directly after cutting the tissue, it is possible to store the dried sections for several days at 4°C. It is recommended to store the microscopic slides in a slide box to avoid condensed water during adaptation to room temperature. Warming up to room temperature requires about 15 min. If the sec-

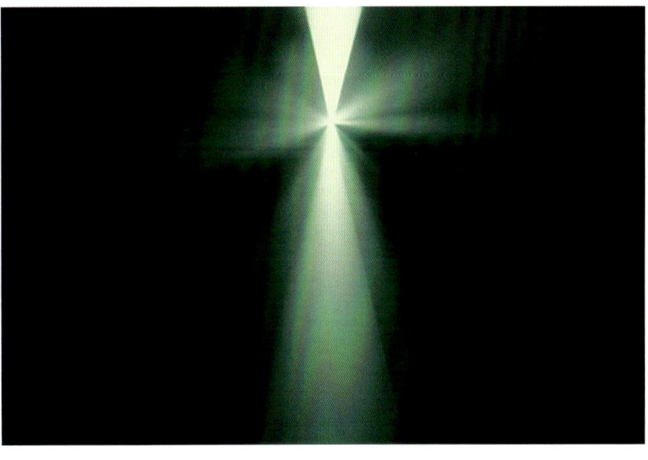

Fig. 92. Laser focus cutting a tissue section. Objective $\times$32; $\times$6.8.

tions have to be stored for months, they must be sealed in plastic foil and stored at –25°C. When the sections are to be used, it is advisable to transfer them first to a 4°C refrigerator and continue as recommended above. A great risk of storing unprocessed cryostat sections at –25°C is the development of ice crystals which destroy the section.

Uncounterstained dehydrogenase and AChE reactions must be fixed in 4% formaldehyde for at least 15 min. A shorter time of fixation denatures tissue sections incompletely and CO_2 gas bubbles are produced in en-

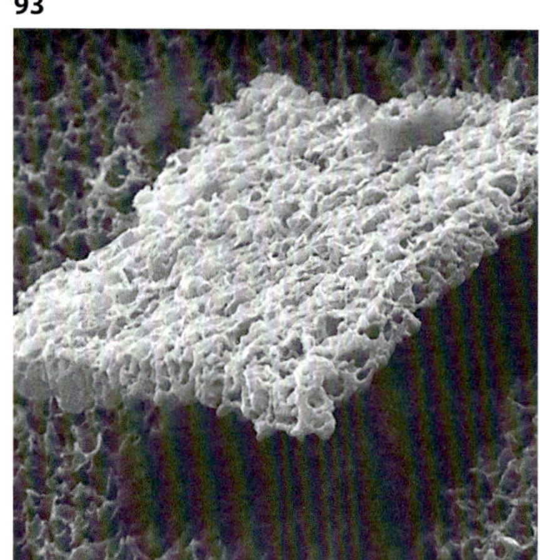

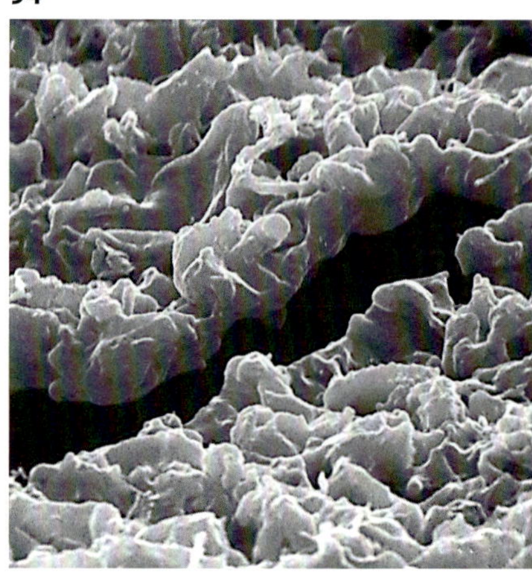

Fig. 93. Laser-prepared rectangular tissue piece of a 15-μm-thick freeze-dried cryostat section. Scanning electron microscope. ×1,000.

Fig. 94. Laser preparation line of a 15-μm-thick freeze-dried cryostat section. Scanning electron microscope. ×5,000.

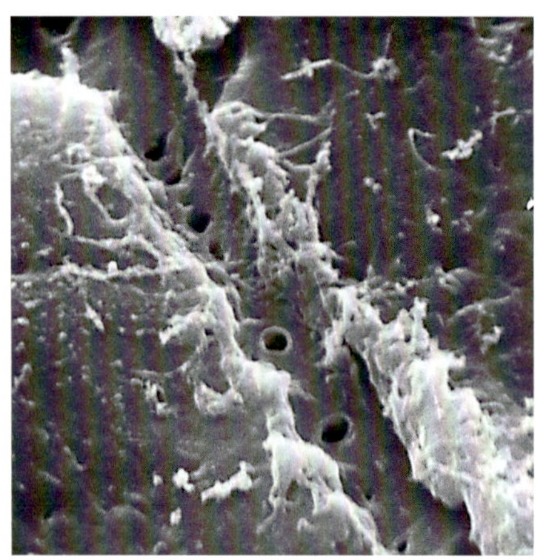

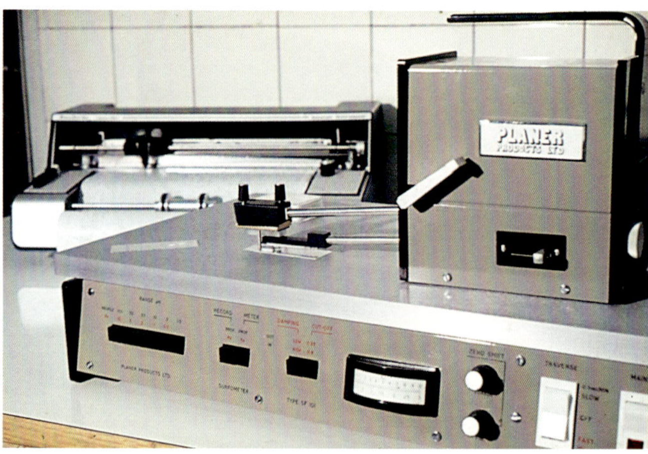

Fig. 95. Laser preparation line of an initial 15-μm thick cryostat section: thawed, spread, and air-dried on a microscopic slide with a notable loss (70%) in section thickness (compare with fig. 94). Scanning electron microscope. ×5,000.

Fig. 96. Physical measuring device ('Planer') to determine section thickness.

zyme-rich structures, which limit the diagnostic evaluation. After fixation, the sections are rinsed twice in tap water and once in demineralized water.

The fixed tissue sections are dried on a hot plate (+60°C), degreased with xylene or xylene substitute and then coated with a quick-hardening mounting medium and covered with a coverslip.

AChE reactions with hemalum counterstaining are not fixed in formalin. After rinsing the sections in tap water, they are dehydrated in a series of increasing alcohol concentrations. After 95% alcohol, the sections are stained with hemalum. After bluing in warm tap water, the wet sections are covered with Crystal/Mount® (Bio-

meda, Foster City, Calif., USA) and dried at 70°C on a hot plate. This procedure stabilizes the hemalum staining which would otherwise fade in 1 to 2 weeks. The diagnostic evaluation of an AChE reaction is performed in uncounterstained sections.

Histopathology of Chonic Constipation

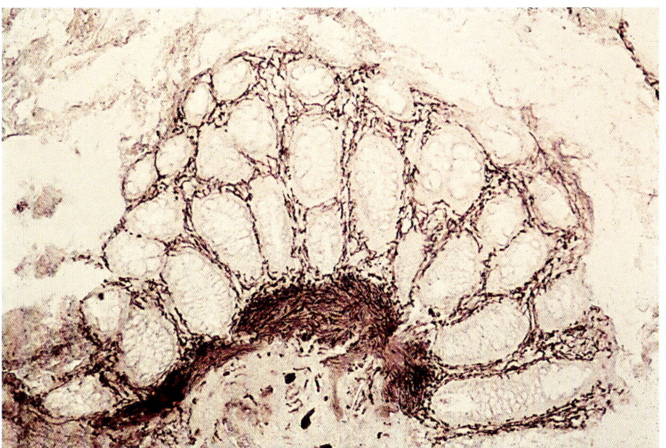

Fig. 97. HD with increased AChE activity in parasympathetic nerves of lamina propria mucosae und muscularis mucosae (8-month-old boy). ×45.

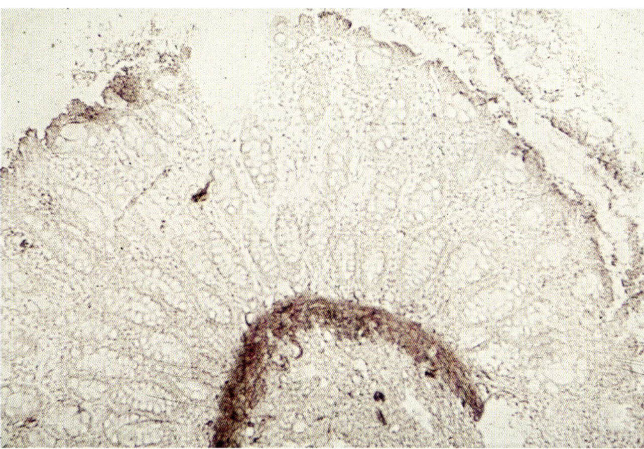

Fig. 98. AChE reaction of normal innervated rectum mucosa (1-year-old boy). ×45.

Preparation of Incubation Media for the Daily Routine of Enzyme Histochemical Reactions

General Remarks: To eliminate the influence of subjective variation in the preparation of incubation media for enzyme histochemical reactions, it is advisable to prepare stock media according to the expected incubations in a 6- to 9-month period.

Processing of Stock Media for Storage at –25°C

1 Prepare 1,000–2,000 ml of medium which may be sufficient for 6–9 months.
2 Bottle the medium in sealed plastic bottles each containing 30–40 ml of medium. This amount may be sufficient for the incubation of 15 microscopic slides in a Hellendahl vessel.
3 Freeze and store at –20 to –30°C.

Handling of Frozen Incubation Medium

1 Frozen medium is thawed in hot tap water (about 40°C).
2 Bring medium to required incubation temperature of 37°C.
3 Cloudy medium has no influence on the incubation result.

Acetylcholinesterase Reaction Medium

The incubation medium (A and B) is thawed and mixed before use (tables 1, 2). AChE demonstrates the cholinergic nervous system. Incubation is at 37°C for 90 min. Parasympathetic structures such as nerve fibers and ganglia are stained brown [209]. The results can be seen in figures 97 and 98.

Table 1. AChE incubation medium A

		100 ml	1,000 ml
(1)	Sodium acetate · 3 H_2O, g	0.514	5.14
(2)	Trisodium citrate · 2 H_2O, g	0.143	1.43
(3)	Copper sulfate · H_2O, g	0.075	0.75
(4)	Acetylthiocholine iodide, g	0.050	0.50
(5)	Distilled water, ml	90	900
(6)	Iso-OMPA, g[1]	0.003	0.03

[1] Tetraisopropyl pyrophosphoramide; Sigma Ltd., inhibitor of nonspecific esterase.

Table 2. AChE incubation medium B

		100 ml	1,000 ml
(1)	Potassium ferricyanide, g	0.016	0.165
(2)	Distilled water, ml	10	100

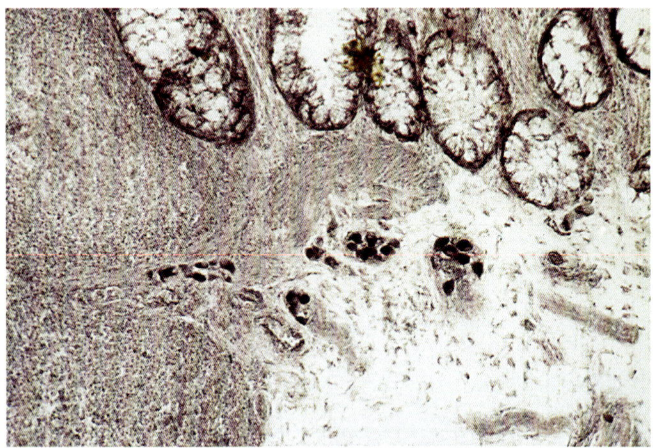

Fig. 99. LDH staining of nerve cells in ganglia of submucous plexus. ×80.

Fig. 100. SDH reaction of mature nerve cells. ×48.

Lactic Dehydrogenase Reaction Medium

LDH intensively stains nerve cells and arterial vessels. It is important to differentiate small arterial vessels from nerve cells. It is helpful to identify the unstained nucleus of nerve cells. LDH stains cytoplasma of nerve cells and smooth muscles. Incubation is at 37°C in a shaking bath for 8–10 min. If the reaction is weak, prolong incubation time. It is advisable to add 2 ml of TNBT (tetranitro blue tetrazolium chloride; 250 mg of TNBT in 10 ml of N,N-dimethylformamide) to the thawed medium. Table 3 shows the LDH incubation medium and table 4 details an alternate buffer in case no commercial phosphate buffer is available. No influence on reaction is expected if the medium becomes cloudy [210]. The result can be seen in figure 99.

Succinic Dehydrogenase Reaction Medium

SDH is a mitochondrial enzyme. Immature nerve cells, due to a deficiency of trophic factors, show a low SDH activity (fig. 101). Immature nerve cells are characterized by a low number of small-sized mitochondria [211]. Mature nerve cells are stained with the same intensity as LDH-positive nerve cells. TNBT in dimethylformamide must be given slowly to the medium by a dropper. Medium may be stirred by an electromagnetic stirrer. It may be helpful to give 0.005 g of β-nicotinamide adenine DL-nucleotide reduced form (NADH) to the thawed medium as an activator of the enzyme reaction. Also, 2 ml of TNBT may be added to the 37°C warmed medium. Incubation needs 8–10 min in a shaking bath (table 5) [212]. The results can be seen in figures 100 and 101.

Table 3. LDH incubation medium

	100 ml	1,000 ml
(1) PBS phosphate buffer (0.01 M; pH 7.4), ml	100	1,000
(2) Sodium *l*-lactate, g	1.120	11.20
(3) Sodium cyanide (adjusted with 1 *N* HCl to pH 7.4), g	0.050	0.50
(4) Magnesium chloride · 6 H_2O, g	0.101	1.01
(5) TNBT, ml[1]	0.5	5.0

Before the medium is applied to the cryostat sections, 0.1 g of β-nicotinamide adenine dinucleotide is added to the medium to start the LDH reaction and 0.005 g of reduced β-nicotinamide adenine-DL-nucleotide (NADH) is given as an activator.

[1] Stock solution: 250 mg of TNBT dissolved in 5 ml of N,N-dimethylformamide.

Table 4. Alternate buffer

Na_2HPO_4 · 2 H_2O stock solution (11.87 g/1,000 ml)	61.2	612
KH_2PO_4 stock solution (9.08 g/1,000 ml)	38.8	388

Nitroxide Synthase Reaction Medium (NADH Diaphorase)

NOS is an unspecific nerve cell marker which stains even immature nerve cells. It is a quick-running simple reaction [213]. NOS is used to stain nerve cells in the proximal resection margin of a resected distal colon to

Table 5. SDH incubation medium

	100 ml	1,000 ml
(1) PBS phosphate buffer (0.01 M; pH 7.4), ml[1]	90	900
(2) Sodium succinate, g	2.7	27
(3) Adjust medium with distilled water, ml	10	100
(4) TNBT, ml[2]	0.5	5

[1] If no commercial phosphate buffer is available, prepare buffer as described in the prescription of LDH medium.
[2] Stock solution: 250 mg of TNBT dissolved in 5 ml of N,N-dimethylformamide.

Table 6. NOS incubation medium

	100 ml	1,000 ml
(1) PBS phosphate buffer (0.01 M; pH 7.4), ml[1]	100	1,000
(2) TNBT, ml[2]	0.5	5

The dry cryostat sections must previously be fixed for 13 min in a 0.4% ice-cold (4°C) paraformaldehyde solution (4 g of paraformaldehyde/1,000 ml phosphate buffer, pH 7.4). Paraformaldehyde needs 24 h to dissolve. The solution is stored at 4°C. This fixation decreases background staining and nerve cells become more distinct and visible. Before the medium is applied to the sections, 0.01 g of reduced β-nicotinamide adenine-DL-nucleotide (NADH) is adjusted.

[1] If no commercial phosphate buffer is available, prepare phosphate buffer as described in the preparation of LDH medium.
[2] Stock solution: 250 mg of TNBT dissolved in 5 ml N,N-dimethylformamide.

exclude aganglionosis, hypoganglionosis, or nerve cell hypoplasia. NOS is an important reaction if a microscopic examination under surgery is necessary. No paraformaldehyde fixation is performed under this condition. A diagnosis can be made after 5 to 6 min of incubation (table 6).

A so-called rapid AChE reaction [34–37, 52] is not very helpful for the control of innervation in the proximal resection line. The caudocranial decrease of the nerve fiber density from the sacral roots S2–S4 (fig. 8) in aganglionosis has the risk of misinterpretation of the innervation pattern (fig. 10). The results can be seen in figures 102 and 103.

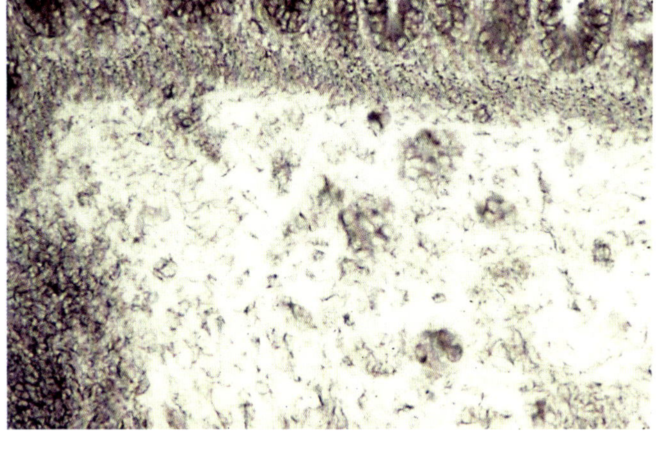

Fig. 101. Submucous plexus with immature ganglia. SDH reaction. ×48.

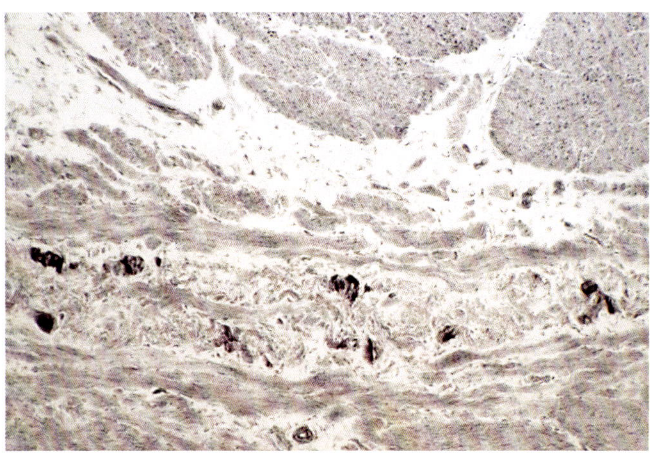

Fig. 102. NOS reaction of heterotopic myenteric plexus. ×120.

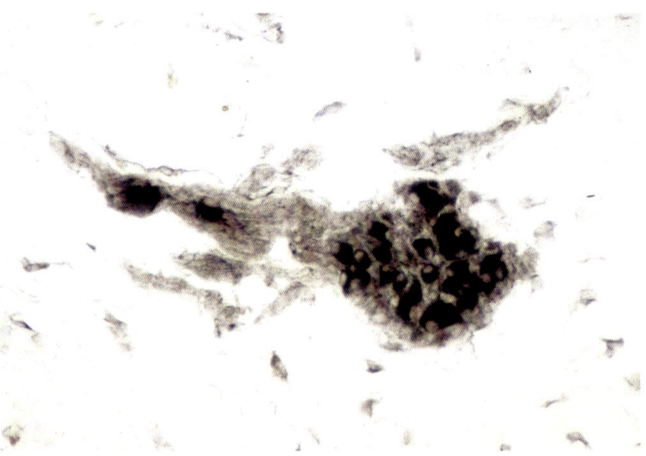

Fig. 103. NOS reaction of a giant ganglion in submucosa. ×440.

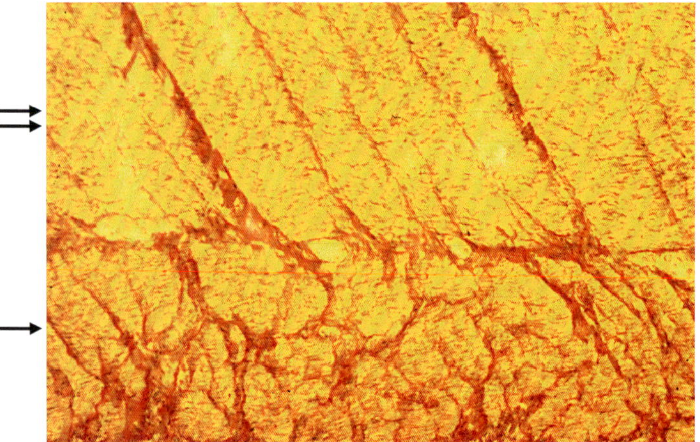

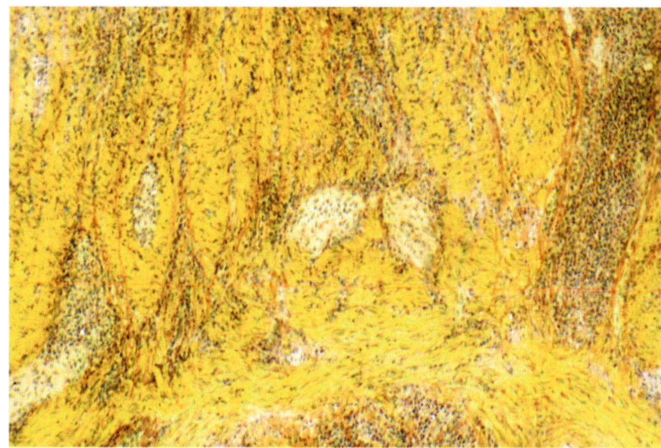

Fig. 104. Normal tendinous net in longitudinal (arrow) and circular muscles (double arrow). Cutting angle 45°. ×180.

Fig. 105. Crohn's disease with destruction of all collagen structures (atrophic desmosis) in circular and longitudinal muscles (compare with fig. 104). Picrosirius red staining. ×180.

Picrosirius Red Staining of Collagen Structures

Picrosirius red staining has proven to be the best differentiating staining of connective tissue versus smooth muscles of the gut (fig. 104, 105). Cryostat sections are first fixed for 45 min in Delaunay fixative: 500 ml of absolute alcohol; 500 ml of acetone; 20 ml of 1 M trichloroacetic acid solution in demineralized water.

Trichloroacetic acid deteriorates time dependently and may be adjusted after 5 weeks. If trichloroacetic acid is no longer effective, smooth muscles are stained red instead of yellow. After Delaunay fixation, sections are stained for 5–10 min in a celestine blue solution.

Preparation of Celestine Blue Solution

The celestine blue mixture [22.5 g of ammonium iron III sulfate dodecahydrate (iron alum), 240 ml of aqua dest., 2.25 g of celestine blue] must be cooked (5–8 min). The solution produces a lot of foam when cooking, but this can be limited by stirring (use a big vessel). Foam slowly disappears during cooking. The solution is cooled to room temperature, filtered, and mixed with 63 ml of glycerol.

Celestine blue solution shows a time-dependent fading of staining intensity, which can be compensated in the beginning by increasing staining time. Residue of the celestine blue solution on the microscopic slides may be eliminated by cellulose wadding. Afterwards, Shandon® hemalum grade 3 staining is performed for 5 min.

Sections are rinsed in warm tap water for bluing. Residue of celestine blue solution deteriorates over time the hemalum solution. A 40-min picrosirius red staining follows the staining of the cell nuclei.

Preparation of Picrosirius Red Solution

Dissolve 0.1 g of sirius red in 500 ml of saturated picric acid solution (15 g of picric acid in 950 ml of aqua dest.). It is recommended to have a small amount of picric acid crystals at the bottom of the sirius red solution vessel to guarantee that the picric acid is always saturated.

Collagen stains red and smooth muscles stain yellow. In comparison to van Gieson or trichrome staining, picrosirius red produces a brilliant contrast. Picrosirius red solution is very stable. The results can be seen in figures 104 and 105.

Histopathology of Chonic Constipation

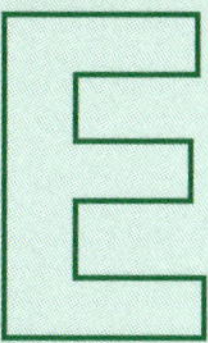

Immunohistochemical Techniques of Paraffin Sections in the Diagnosis of Gut Dysmotility

Immunohistochemistry must be used in formalin-fixed paraffin-embedded biopsies or surgical specimens. In comparison to enzyme histochemistry, immunohistochemistry has a series of limitations. These include:

1 Immunohistochemistry is not as reliable as enzyme histochemistry and is a static technique like hemalum/eosin staining.
2 Aganglionosis of the anal ring or the distal rectum mucosa (ultrashort HD) cannot be reliably diagnosed by immunohistochemical means.
3 Immunohistochemistry needs more time from taking the biopsy to diagnosis than enzyme histochemistry, and it is not as cheap.
4 No opportunity to examine the proximal resection line during surgery.

The following tissue compartments of the intestinal wall can be stained by immunohistochemical means:

Nerve cells:
- Cathepsin D with osmium tetroxide contrasting [148, 149]
- MAP 2 (microtubule-associated protein) [147, 214]
- PGP 9.5 [215]

Glial cells:
- S100

Nerve fibers:
- Calretinin (negative reaction of nerve fibers in mucosa in aganglionosis) [216, 217].

It is not possible to evaluate functional consequences with a low nerve cell number, immaturity of the enteral nervous system, or hypoplasia of nerve cells diagnosed by an immunohistochemical observation. Enzyme histochemistry allows a prognosis of colonic function of hypoganglionosis or any other dysganglionosis [218].

References

1 Bruder E: Gastrointestinal motility disorders. Interdisciplinary presentation of a complex disease (in German). Pathologe 2007;28:92–172.
2 Meier-Ruge WA, Bruder E: Pathology of chronic constipation in pediatric and adult coloproctology. Pathobiology 2005;72:1–102.
3 Meier-Ruge W: On the pathology and bioptic diagnosis of Hirschsprung's disease in relation to acquired and functional megacolon (in German). Verh Dtsch Ges Pathol 1967;51:323–328.
4 Meier-Ruge WA, Bruder E: Histopathology of ultrashort Hirschsprung's disease and aganglionic musculus corrugator cutis ani. Pathobiology 2005;72:26–29.
5 Meier-Ruge W, Lutterbeck PM, Herzog B, Morger R, Moser R, Schärli A: Acetylcholinesterase activity in suction biopsies of the rectum in the diagnosis of Hirschsprung's disease. J Pediatr Surg 1972;7:11–17.
6 Goto S, Ikeda K, Toyohara T: Histochemical confirmation of the acetylcholinesterase-activity in rectal suction biopsy from neonates with Hirschsprung's disease. Z Kinderchir 1984;39:246–249.
7 Heitz PU, Komminoth P: Biopsy diagnosis of Hirschsprung's disease and related disorders. Curr Top Pathol 1990;81:257–275.
8 Nakao M, Suita S, Taguchi T, Hirose R, Shima Y: Fourteen-year experience of acetylcholinesterase staining for rectal mucosal biopsy in neonatal Hirschsprung's disease. J Pediatr Surg 2001;36:1357–1363.
9 Meier-Ruge WA, Bruder E: Current concepts of enzyme histochemistry in modern pathology. Pathobiology 2008;75:233–243.
10 Pearse AG: Histochemistry: Theoretical and Applied, ed 2. London, J & A Churchill, 1960.
11 Pearse AG: Histochemistry: Theoretical and Applied, ed 3. London, Churchill Livingstone, 1968.
12 Lojda Z, Gossrau R, Schiebler TH: Enzyme Histochemistry. A Laboratory Manual. Berlin, Springer, 1979.
13 Meier-Ruge WA, Bruder E: Histopathology of Hirschsprung disease; in Nunez R, Lopez-Alonso M (eds): Hirschsprung's Disease: Diagnosis and Treatment. Hauppage, Nova Science Publishers Inc, 2009, pp 107–121.
14 Virchow R: Ueber die Standpunkte in der wissenschaftlichen Medizin. Virchows Arch 1867;1:5–19.
15 Virchow R: Die wissenschaftliche Methode und die Standpunkte in der Therapie. Virchows Arch 1869;2:3–37.
16 Bruder A, Meier-Ruge W: Zur Pathologie des Hirninfarktes unter besonderer Berücksichtigung der frühen Stadien einer hypoxischen Ischaemie. Geriatrie Rehabilitation 1990;3:53–85.
17 Meier-Ruge W, Bruder A, Theodore D: Histochemical and morphometric investigation of the pathogenesis of acute brain infarction in primates. Acta Histochem Suppl 1992;42:59–70.
18 Meier-Ruge W, Theodore D, Abraham J: Pathology of ischemic brain damage – implication for therapy; in Somjen G (ed): Cerebral Hypoxia and Stroke. New York, Plenum Press, 1988, pp 73–81.
19 Feichter S, Meier-Ruge WA, Bruder E: The histopathology of gastrointestinal motility disorders in children. Semin Pediatr Surg 2009;18:206–211.
20 Bruder E, Meier-Ruge WA: Twenty years diagnostic competence center for Hirschsprung's disease in Basel (in German). Chirurg 2010;81:572–576.
21 Knowles CH, De Giorgio R, Kapur RP, Bruder E, et al: Gastrointestinal neuromuscular pathology: guidelines for histological techniques and reporting on behalf of the Gastro 2009 International Working Group. Acta Neuropathol 2009;118:271–301.
22 Meier-Ruge W, Bruder E: Histopathological diagnosis and differential diagnosis of Hirschsprung disease; in Holschneider AM, Puri P (eds): Hirschsprung's Disease and Allied Disorders. Berlin, Springer, 2008, pp 185–197.
23 Santos MM, Tannuri U, Coelho MC: Study of actelycholinesterase activity in rectal suction biopsy for diagnosis of intestinal dysganglionoses: 17-year experience of a single center. Pediatr Surg Int 2008;24:715–719.
24 Montedonico S, Piotriowska AP, Rolle U, Puri P: Histochemical staining of rectal suction biopsies as the first investigation in patients with chronic constipation. Pediatr Surg Int 2008;24:785–792.
25 de Brito IA, Maksoud JG: Evolution with age of the acetylcholinesterase activity in rectal suction biopsy in Hirschsprung's disease. J Pediatr Surg 1987;22:425–430.

26 Meier-Ruge WA, Bruder E: Characteristics of Hirschsprung's disease. Pathobiol 2005;72:10–21.

27 Coelho MC, Tannuri U, Benditt I, Santos MM: Studies of RET gene expression and acetylcholinesterase activity in a series of sporadic Hirschsprung's disease. Pediatr Surg Int 2008;24:1017–1021.

28 Tomita R, Munakata K, Howard ER, Fujisaki S: Histological studies on Hirschsprung's disease and its allied disorders in childhood. Hepatogastroenterology 2004;51:1042–1044.

29 Meier-Ruge W: Das Megacolon. Seine Diagnose und Pathophysiologie. Virchows Arch A Pathol Pathol Anat 1968;344:67–85.

30 Park WH, Choi SO, Kwon KY, Chang ES: Acetylcholinesterase histochemistry of rectal suction biopsies in the diagnosis of Hirschsprung's disease. J Korean Med Sci 1992;7:353–359.

31 Coffin CM, Spilker K, Zhou H, Lowichik A, Pysher TJ: Frozen section diagnosis in pediatric surgical pathology: a decade's experience in a children's hospital. Arch Pathol Lab Med 2005;129:1619–1625.

32 Moore SW, Johnson G: Acetylcholesterase in Hirschsprung's disease. Pediatr Surg Int 2005;21:255–263.

33 Meier-Ruge WA, Bruder E: Preparation of cryostat sections from biopsies and colorectal specimens. Pathobiology 2005;72:93–94.

34 Kobayashi H, O'Briain DS, Hirakawa H Wang Y, Puri P: A rapid technique of acetylcholesterase staining. Ach Pathol Lab Med 1994;118:1127–1129.

35 Kobayashi H, Wang Y, Hirakawa H, O'Briain, Puri P: Intraoperative evaluation of extent of aganglionosis by a rapid acetylcholinesterase histochemical technique. J Pediatr Surg 1995;30:248–252.

36 Meyrat BJ, Lesbros Y, Laurini RN: Assessment of the colon innervation with serial biopsies above the aganglionic zone before the pull-through procedure in Hirschsprung's disease. Pediatr Surg Int 2001;17:129–135.

37 Martucciello G, Favre A, Torre M, Pini Prato A, Jasonni V: A new rapid acetylcholinesterase histochemical method for the intraoperative diagnosis of Hirschsprung's disease and intestinal neuronal dysplasia. Eur J Pediatr Surg 2001;11:300–304.

38 Kapur RP: Practical pathology and genetics of Hirschsprung's disease. Semin Pediatr Surg 2009;18:212–223.

39 Martucciello G, Ceccherini I, Lerone M, Jasonni V: Pathogenesis of Hirschsprung's Disease. J Pediatr Surg 2000;35:1017–1025.

40 Amiel J, Lyonnet S: Hirschsprung disease, associated syndromes, and genetics: a review. J Med Genet 2001;38:729–739.

41 Meier-Ruge WA, Bruder E: Total aganglionosis of the colon. Pathobiology 2005;72:19–23.

42 Choe EK, Moon SB, Kim HY, Lee SC, Park KW, Jung SE: Outcomes of surgical management of total aganglionosis. World J Surg 2008;32:62–68.

43 Moore SW, Zaahl M: Clinical and genetic differences in total aganglionosis in Hirschsprung's disease. J Pediatr Surg 2009;44:1899–1903.

44 Sakai T, Nirasawa Y, Itoh Y, Wakizaka A: Japanese patients with sporadic Hirschsprung: mutation analysis of the receptor tyrosine kinase proto-oncogene, endothelin-B receptor, endothelin-3, glial cell line-derived neurotrophic factor and neurturin genes: a comparison with similar studies. Eur J Pediatr 2000;159:160–167.

45 Garcia-Barcelo M, Sham MH, Lee WS, Lui VC, Chen BL, Wong KK, Wong JS, Tam PK: Highly recurrent RET mutations and novel mutations in genes of the receptor tyrosine kinase and endothelin receptor B pathways in Chinese patients with sporadic Hirschsprung disease. Clin Chem 2004;50:93–100.

46 Kapur RP: Hirschsprung disease and other enteric dysganglionoses. Crit Rev Clin Lab Sci 1999;36:225–273.

47 Parisi MA, Kapur RP: Genetics of Hirschsprung disease. Curr Opin Pediatr 200;12:610–617.

48 Amiel J, Sproat-Emison E, Garcia-Barcelo M, Lantieri F, Burzynski S et al: Hirschsprung disease, associated syndromes and genetics: a review. J Med Genet 2008;45:1–14.

49 de Pontual L, Zaghloul NA, Thomas S, Davis EE, Mc Gaughey DM, et al: Epistasis between RET and BBS mutations modulates enteric innervation and causes syndromic Hirschsprung disease. Proc Natl Acad Sci USA 2009;106:13921–13926.

50 Lantieri F, Griseri P, Ceccherini I: Molecular mechanisms of RET-induced Hirschsprung pathogenesis. Ann Med 2006;38:11–19.

51 Emison ES, Garcia-Barcelo M, Grice EA, Lantieri F, Amiel J, et al: Differential contribution of rare and common, coding and noncoding RET mutations to multifactorial Hirschsprung disease liability. Am J Hum Genet 2010;87:60–74.

52 Moore SW, Johnson AG: Hirschsprung's disease: genetic and functional associations of Down's and Waardenburg syndromes. Semin Pediatr Surg 1998;7:156–161.

53 Inoue K, Ohyama T, Sakuragi Y, Yamamoto R, Inoue NA, et al: Translation of SOX10 3′ untranslated region causes a complex severe neurocristopathy by generation of a deleterious functional domain. Hum Mol Genet 2007;16:3037–3046.

54 Tüysüz B, Collin A, Arapoglu M, Suyugül N: Clinical variability of Waardenburg-Shah syndrome in patients with proximal 13q deletion syndrome including the endothelin-B receptor locus. Am J Med Genet A 2009;149A:2290–2295.

55 Pingault V, Ente D, Dastot-Le Moal F, Goossens W, Martin S, Bondurand N: Review and update of mutations causing Waardenburg syndrome. Hum Mutat 2010;31:391–406.

56 Verheij FB, Sival DA, van der Hoeven JH, Vos YJ, Meiners LC, Brouwer CF, van Essens AJ: Shah-Waardenburg syndrome and PCWH associated with SOX10 mutations: a case report and review of the literature. Eur J Peadiatr Neurol 2006;10:11–17.

57 Shimotake T, Tanaka S, Fukui R, Makino S, Maruyama R: Neuroglial disorders of central and peripheral nervous systems in a patient with Hirschsprung's disease carrying allelic SOX10 truncating mutation. J Pediatr Surg 2007;42:725–731.

58 Mowat DR, Wilson MJ, Goossens M: Mowat-Wilson syndrome. J Med Genet 2003;40:305–310.

59 Zweier C, Thiel CT, Dufke A, Crow YJ, Meinecke P, Suri M, et al: Clinical and mutational spectrum of Mowat-Wilson syndrome. Eur J Med Genet 2005;48:97–111.

60 Ridanpää M, van Eenennaam H, Pelin K, Chadwick R, Johnson C, et al: Mutations in the RNA component of RNase MRP cause a pleiotropic human disease, cartilage-hair hypoplasia. Cell 2001;104:195–203.

61 Mäkitie O, Kaitila I, Rintala R: Hirschsprung disease associated with severe cartilage-hair hypoplasia. J Pediatr 2001;138:929–931.

62 Moolenbeek C, Rutenberg EJ: The 'Swiss roll': a simple technique for histological studies of the rodent intestine. Lab Anim 1962,15:57–59.

63 Mastracci L, Bruno S, Spaggiari P, Ceppa P, Fiocca R: The impact of biopsy number and site on the accuracy of intestinal metaplasia detection in the stomach. A morphometric study based on virtual biopsies. Dig Liver Dis 2008;40:632–640.

64 Osterheld MC, Meagher-Villemure K, Ciola AM, Martin P, Vilasa D, Meyrat BJ: Hirschsprung's disease: the 'Swiss roll' technique revisited. Pediatr Surg Int 2009;25:573–578.

65 Meier-Ruge WA, Bruder E: Methodology of enzyme histochemistry in coloproctological motility disorders. Pathobiology 2005;72:91–99.

66 Meier-Ruge WA, Brunner LA, Engert J, Heminghaus M, Holschneuider AM, et al: A correlative morphometric and clinical investigation of hypoganglionosis of the colon in children. Eur J Pediatr Surg 1999;9:67–74.

67 Meier-Ruge WA, Brunner LA: Morphometric assessment of Hirschsprung's disease: associated hypoganglionosis of the colonic myenteric plexus. Pediatr Dev Pathol 2001;4:53–61.

68 Maia DM: The reliability of frozen-section diagnosis in the pathologic evaluation of Hirschsprung's disease. Am J Surg Pathol 2000;24:1675–1677.

69 Shayan K, Smith C, Langer JC: Reliability of intraoperative frozen sections in the management of Hirschsprung's disease. J Pediatr Surg 2004;39:1345–1348.

70 Boman F, Sfeir R, Priso R, Bonnevalle M, Besson R: Advantages of intraoperative semiquantitative evaluation of myenteric nervous plexus in patients with Hirschsprung disease. J Pediatr Surg 2007;42:1089–1094.

71 Das K, Kini U, Babu MK, Mohanty S, D'Cruz AJ: The distal level of normally innervated bowel in long segment colonic Hirschsprung's disease. Pediatr Surg Int 2010;26:593–599.

72 Meier-Ruge W, Schärli AF: The epidemiology and enzyme histochemical characterization of ultrashort-segment Hirschsprung's disease. Pediatr Surg Int 1986;1:37–42.

73 Meier-Ruge WA, Bruder E, Holschneider AM, Lochbühler H, Piket G, Posselt HG, Tewes G: Diagnosis and therapy of ultrashort Hirschsprung's disease. Eur J Pediatr Surg 2004;14:392–397.

74 Ballard ET: Ultrashort segment Hirschsprung's disease: a case report. Pediatr Pathol Lab Med 1996;16:319–325.

75 Bruder E, Teracciano LM, Passarge E, Meier-Ruge WA: Enzyme histochemistry of classical and ultrashort Hirschsprung's disease (in German). Pathologe 2007;28:105–112.

76 Bagdzevicius R, Vaicekauskas V, Bagdzeviciute S: Experience of acetylcholinesterase histochemistry application in the diagnosis of chronic constipation in children. Medicina (Kaunas) 2007;43:376–384.

77 Holschneider AM: Anal sphincter achalasia and ultrashort Hirschsprung's disease; in Holschneider AM, Puri P (eds): Hirschsprung's Disease and Allied Disorders, ed 2. Amsterdam, Harwood Acad Publ, 2000, pp 399–424.

78 Scobie WG, Mackinlay GA: Anorectal myectomy in treatment of ultrashort segment Hirschsprung's disease. Arch Dis Child 1977;52:713–715.

79 Shermeta DW, Nilprabhassorn P: Posterior myectomy for primary and secondary short segment aganglionosis. Am J Surg 1977;133:39–41.

80 Sauvat F, Grimaldi C, Lacaille F, Ruemmele F, et al: Intestinal transplantation for total intestinal aganglionosis: a series of 12 consecutive children. J Pediatr Surg 2008;43:1833–1838.

81 Lao OB, Healey PJ, Perkins JD, Reyes JD, Goldin AB: Outcomes in children with intestinal failure following listing for intestinal transplant. J Pediatr Surg 2010;45:100–107.

82 Tsuji H, Spitz L, Kiely EM, Drake DP, Pierro A: Management and long-term follow-up of infants with total colonic aganglionosis. J Pediatr Surg 1999;34:158–161.

83 Wildhaber BE, Teitelbaum DH, Coran AG: Total colonic Hirschsprung's disease: a 28-year experience. J Pediatr Surg 2005;40:203–206.

84 Anupama B, Zheng S, Xiao X: Ten-year experience in the management of total colonic aganglionosis. J Pediatr Surg 2007;42:1671–1676.

85 Leiri S, Suita S, Nakatsuji T, Akioshi J, Taguchi T: Total colonic aganglionosis with or without small bowel involvement: a 30-year retrospective nationwide survey in Japan. J Pediatr Surg 2008;43:2226–2230.

86 Menezes M, Pini Prato A, Jasonni V, Puri P: Long-term clinical outcome in patients with total colonic aganglionosis: a 31-year review. J Pediatr Surg 2008;43:1696–1699.

87 Shen C, Song Z, Zheng S, Xiao X: A comparison of the effectiveness of the Soave and Martin procedure for the treatment of total colonic aganglionosis. J Pediatr Surg 2009;44:2355–2358.

88 Smith VV: Intestinal neuronal density in childhood: a baseline for the objective assessment of hypo- and hyperganglionosis. Pediatr Pathol 1993;13:225–237.

89 Holschneider AM, Meier-Ruge W: Hirschsprung's disease and allied disorders – a review. Eur J Pediatr Surg 1994;4:260–266.

90 Watanabe Y, Ito F, Ando H, Seo T, et al: Morphological investigation of the enteric nervous system in Hirschsprung's disease and hypoganglionosis using whole-mount colon preparation. J Pediatr Surg 1999;34:445–449.

91 Farrugia MK, Alexander N, Clarke S, Nash R, et al: Does transitional zone pull-through in Hirschsprung's disease imply a poor prognosis? J Pediatr Surg 2003;38:1766–1769.

92 Dübbers M, Holschneider AM, Meier-Ruge W: Results of total and subtotal colon resections in children. Eur J Pediatr Surg 2003;13:195–200.

93 Schulten D, Holschneider AM, Meier-Ruge W: Proximal segment histology of resected bowel in Hirschsprung's disease predicts postoperative bowel function. Eur J Pediatr Surg 2000;10:378–381.

94 Yadav AK, Mishra K, Agarwal S, Mohta A: Role of computerized morphometric analysis in the diagnosis of Hirschsprung's disease. Anal Quant Cytol Histol 2010;32:114–116.

95 Munakata K, Okabe I, Morita K: Clinical and histologic studies of abnormal intramural plexus with special reference to hypoganglionosis (in Japanese). Nippon Geka Gekkai Zasshi 1986;87:200–205.

96 Wedel T, Roblick UJ, Ott V, Eggers R, et al: Oligoneuronal hypoganglionosis in patients with idiopathic slow-transit constipation. Dis Colon Rectum 2002;45:54–62.

97 Tomita R, Munakata K, Howard ER, Fujisaki S: Histological studies on Hirschsprung's disease and its allied disorders in childhood. Hepatogastroenterology 2004;51:1042–1044.

98 Bruder E, Meier-Ruge WA: Hypoganglionosis as a cause of chronic constipation (in German). Pathologe 2007;28:131–136.

99 Thang HY, Feng JX, Huang L, Wang G, et al: Diagnosis and surgical treatment of isolated hypoganglionosis. World J Pediatr 2008;4:295–300.

100 Munakata K, Okabe I, Norita K: Histologic studies of rectocolic aganglionosis and allied diseases. J Pediatr Surg 1978;13:67–75.

101 Howard ER, Garrett JR, Kidd A: Constipation and congenital disorders of the myenteric plexus. J R Soc Med 1984;77:13–19.

102 Schärli AF, Sossai R: Hypoganglionosis. Semin Pediatr Surg 1998;7:187–191.

103 Ippolito C, Segnani, C, De Giorgio R, Blandizzi C, et al: Quantitative evaluation of myenteric ganglion cells in normal human left colon: implications for histopathological analysis. Cell Tissue Res 2009;336:191–201.

104 Swaminathan M, Kapur RP: Counting myenteric ganglion cells in histologic sections: an empirical approach. Hum Pathol 2010;41:1097–1108.

105 Brunner LA: Morphometrische Charakterisierung des Plexus myentericus des Colon bei der isolierten und einer Hirschsprung assoziierten Hypoganglionose des Kindes. Inaug Diss, Univ Basel, 1996.

106 Yamataka A, Miyano T, Urao M, Okazaki T: Distribution of neuromuscular junctions in the bowel affected by hypoganglionosis. J Pediatr Gastroenterol Nutr 1993;16:165–167.

107 O'Donnell AM, Puri P: Hypoganglionic colorectum in the chick embryo: a model of human hypoganglionosis. Pediatr Surg Int 2009;25:885–888.

108 Meier-Ruge WA, Bruder E: Hypoplastic neuronal dysganglionosis in the myenteric plexus. Pathobiology 2005;72:75–77.

109 Kobayashi H, Yamataka A, Lane GJ, Miyano T: Pathophysiology of hypoganglionosis. J Pediatr Gastroenterol Nutr 2002;34:231–235.

110 Kobayashi H, Yamataka A, Lane GJ, Miyano T: Rectal biopsy: what is the optimal procedure? Pediatr Surg Int 2002;18:753–756.

111 Dingemann J, Puri P: Isolated hypoganglionosis: systematic review of a rare intestinal innervation defect. Pediatr Surg Int 2010;26:1111–1115.

112 Gershon MD, Rothmann TP: Enteric glia. Glia 1991;4:195–204.

113 Gershon MD, Chalazonitis A, Rothmann TP: From neural crest to bowel: development of the enteric nervous system. J Neurobiol 1993;24:199–214.

114 Gershon MD: Functional anatomy of the enteric nervous system; in Holschneider AM, Puri P (eds): Hirschsprung's Disease and Allied Disorders. Amsterdam, Harwood Acad Publ, 2000, pp 19–58.

115 Gershon MD, Ratcliffe EM: Developmental biology of the enteric nervous system: pathogenesis of Hirschsprung's disease and other congenital dysmotilities. Semin Pediatr Surg 2004;13:224–235.

116 Stoss F, Meier-Ruge WA, Knecht NA, Müller-Lobeck H, Ammann K: Atrophic hypoganglionosis in the colon of adults with slow-transit constipation: a morphometric histopathological investigation. Eur Surg 2005;37:83–87.

117 Ikeda K, Goto S, Nagasaki A, Taguchi T: Hypogenesis of intestinal ganglion cells: a rare cause of intestinal obstruction simulating aganglionosis. Z Kinderchir 1988;43:52–53.

118 Lassmann G, Kees A, Korner K, Wurnig P: Transient functional obstruction of the colon in neonates: examination of its development by manometry and biopsies. Prog Pediatr Surg 1989;24:202–216.

119 Toyosaka A, Tomimoto Y, Nose K, Seki Y, Okamoto E: Immaturity of the myenteric plexus is the aetiology of meconium ileus without mucoviscidosis: a histopathologic study. Clin Auton Res 1994;4:175–184.

120 Ure BM, Holschneider AM, Schulten D, Meier-Ruge W: Clinical impact of intestinal malformations: a prospective study in 141 patients. Pediatr Surg Int 1997;12:377–382.

121 Miyahara K, Kato Y, Seki T, Arakawa A, Lane GJ, Yamataka A: Neuronal immaturity in normoganglionic colon from cases of Hirschsprung disease, anorectal malformation, and idiopathic constipation. J Pediatr Surg 2009;44:2364–2368.

122 Meier-Ruge WA, Bruder E: Immaturity of the enteric nervous system. Pathobiology 2005;72:34–36.

123 Erdohazi M: Retarded development of the enteric nerve cells. Dev Med Child Neurol 1974;16:365–368.

124 Meier-Ruge WA, Bruder E: Necrotizing enterocolitis. Pathobiology 2005;72:56–58.

125 Meier-Ruge WA: Idiopathic megacolon. New findings on histopathology and musculo-mechanical causes (in German). Chirurg 2000;71: 927–931.

126 Casuistic of colon disorder with symptoms of Hirschsprung's disease. Verh Dtsch Ges Pathol 1971;55:506–510.

127 Meier-Ruge WA, Longo-Bauer CH: Morphometric determination of the methodological criteria for the diagnosis of intestinal neuronal dysplasia (IND B). Pathol Res Pract 1997;193:465–469.

128 Meier-Ruge WA, Bruder E, Kapur RP: Intestinal neuronal dysplasia type B: one giant ganglion is not good enough. Pediatr Dev Pathol 2006;9:444–452.

129 Coerdt W, Michel JS, Rippin G, Kletzki S, et al: Quantitative morphometric analysis of the submucous plexus in age-related control groups. Virchows Arch 2004;444:239–246.

130 Bruder E, Meier-Ruge W: Intestinal neuronal dysplasia type B: how do we understand it today (in German)? Pathologe 2007;28:137–142.

131 Puri P, Wester T: Intestinal neuronal dysplasia. Semin Pediatr Surg 1998;7:181–186.

132 Schmittenbecheer PP, Sacher P, Cholewa D, Haberlik A, et al: Hirschsprung's disease and intestinal neuronal dysplasia – a frequent association with implications for postoperative course. Pediatr Surg Int 1999;15:553–558.

133 Wilder-Smith CH, Talbot C, Merki HS, Meier-Ruge WA: Morphometric quantification of normal submucous plexus in the distal rectum of adult healthy volunteers. Eur J Gastroenterol Hepatol 2002;14: 1339–1342.

134 Schimpl G, Uray E, Ratschek M, Höllwarth WE: Constipation and intestinal neuronal dysplasia type B: a clinical follow-up study. J Pediatr Gastroenterol Nutr 2004;38:308–311.

135 Munakata K, Morita K, Okabe I, Sueoka H: Clinical and histologic studies of neuronal intestinal dysplasia. J Pediatr Surg 1985;20:231–235.

136 Kapur RP, Correa H: Architectural malformation of the muscularis propria as a cause for intestinal pseudo-obstruction: two cases and a review of the literature. Pediatr Dev Pathol 2009;12:156–164.

137 Martucciello G, Torre M, Pini Prato A, Lerone M, et al: Associated anomalies in intestinal neuronal dyplasia. J Pediatr Surg 2002;37:219–223.

138 Skaba R, Meier-Ruge W, Dudorkinova D: Disseminated intestinal hypoganglionosis treated by colectomy and tapering of the small intestine. A case report. Eur J Pediatr Surg 2002;12:203–208.

139 Corduk N, Koltuksuz U, Bir F, Karabul M, et al: Association of rare intestinal malformations: colonic atresia and intestinal neuronal dysplasia. Adv Ther 2007;24:1254–1259.

140 Gath R, Goessling A, Keller KM, Koletzko S, et al: Analysis of the RET, GDNF, EDN3, and EDNRB genes in patients with intestinal neuronal dysplasia and Hirschsprung disease. Gut 2001;48:671–675.

141 Fava M, Borghini S, Cinti R, Cusano R, et al: HOX11L1: a promotor study to evaluate possible expression defects in intestinal motility disorders. Int J Mol Med 2000;10:101–108.

142 von Boyen GB, Krammer HJ, Süss A, Dembowski C, et al: Abnormalities of the enteric nervous system in heterozygous endothelin B receptor deficient (spotting lethal) rats resembling intestinal neuronal dysplasia. Gut 2002;51:414–419.

143 Holland-Cunz S, Krammer HJ, Süss A, Tafazzoli K, et al: Molecular genetics of colorectal motility disorders. Eur J Pediatr Surg 2003;13: 146–151.

144 Skaba R, Frantlova M, Horak J: Intestinal neuronal dysplasia. Eur J Gastroenterol Hepatol 2006;18:699–701.

145 Guo X, Feng J, Wang G: Anorectal electromanometrical patterns in children with isolated neuronal intestinal dysplasia. Eur J Pediatr Surg 2008;18:176–179.

146 Krammer HJ, Meier-Ruge W, Sigge W, Eggers R, et al: Histopathological features of neuronal intestinal dysplasia of the plexus submucosus in whole mounts revealed by immunohistochemistry for PGP 9.5. Eur J Pediatr Surg 1994;4:358–361.

147 Faussone-Pellegrini MS, Martini P, DeFelici M: The cytoskeleton of the myenteric neurons during embryonic life. Anat Embryol 1999; 199:459–469.

148 Abu-Alfa AK, Khan DF, West AB, et al: Cathepsin D in intestinal ganglion cells: a potential aid to diagnosis in suspected Hirschsprung's disease. Am J Surg Pathol 1987;21:201–205.

149 Dzienis-Koronkiewicz E, Debek W, Sulkowska M, Chyczewski I: Suitability of selected markers for identification of elements of the intestinal nervous system. Eur J Pediatr Surg 2002;12:397–401.

150 Stoss F, Riedler L, Meier-Ruge W: Symptoms and diagnosis of neuronal colonic dysplasia in adults. Acta Chir Austriaca 1991;23(suppl 93):28–29.

151 Stoss F, Meier-Ruge W: Experience with neuronal intestinal dysplasia (NID) in adults. Eur J Pediatr Surg 1994;4:298–302.

152 Moore SW, Lang D, Melis J, Cywes S: Secondary effects of prolonged intestinal obstruction on the enteric nervous system in the rat. J Pediatr Surg 1993;28:1196–1199.

153 d'Amore ES, Manivel JC, Pettinato G, Niehans GA, et al: Intestinal ganglioneuromatosis: mucosal and transmural types. A clinicopathologic and immunohistochemical study of six cases. Hum Pathol 1991; 22:276–286.

154 Smith VV, Eng C, Milla PJ: Intestinal ganglioneuromatosis and multiple endocrine neoplasia type 2B: implications for treatment. Gut 1999;45:143–146.

155 Ohyama T, Sato M, Murao K, Kittaka K, et al: A case of multiple endocrine neoplasia type 2B undiagnosed for many years despite its typical phenotype. Endocrine 2001;15:143–146.

156 Wildhaber B, Niggli F, Bergsträsser E, Stallmach T, et al: Paraneoplastic syndromes in ganglioneuroblastoma: contrasting symptoms of constipation and diarrhoea. Eur J Pediatr 2003;162:511–513.

157 Unruh A, Fitze G, Jänig U, Bielack S, et al: Medullary thyroid carcinoma in a 2-month-old male with multiple endocrine neoplasia 2B and symptoms of pseudo-Hirschsprung disease: a case report. J Pediatr Surg 2007;42:1623–1626.

158 Qiao S, Iwashita T, Ichihara M, Murakumo Y, et al: Increased expression of glia cell line-derived neurotrophic factor and neurturin in a case of colon adenocarcinoma associated with diffuse ganglioneuromatosis. Clin Neuropathol 2009;28:105–112.

159 Takahashi M, Iwashita T, Santoro M, Lyonnet S, et al: Co-segregation of MEN2 and Hirschsprung's disease: the same mutation of RET with both gain and loss-of-function? Hum Mut 1999;13:331–336.

160 Romeo G, Ceccherini I, Celli J, Priolo M et al: Association of multiple endocrine neoplasia type 2 and Hirschsprung's disease. J Intern Med 1998;243:515–520.

161 Goertler K: Der konstruktive Bau der menschlichen Darmwand. Gegenbaurs Morph Jahrb 1932;69:329–358.

162 Penman DG, Lilford RJ: The megacystis-microcolon-intestinal hypoperistalsis syndrome: a fatal autosomal recessive condition. J Med Genet 1989;26:66–67.

163 Anneren G, Meurling S, Olsen L: Megacystis-microcolon intestinal hypoperistalsis syndrome (MMIHS), an autosomal recessive disorder: clinical reports and review of the literature. Am J Med Genet 1991; 41:251–254.

164 Chung MY, Huang CB, Chuang JH, Ko SF, et al: Megacystis-microcolon-intestinal hypoperistalsis syndrome (MMIHS): a case report. Changgeng Yi Xue Za Zhi 1998;21:92–96.

165 Moore SW, Schneider JW, Kaschula RO: Unusual variation of gastrointestinal smooth muscle abnormalities associated with chronic intestinal pseudo-obstruction. Pediatr Surg Int 2002;18:13–20.

166 Marshall DG, Meier-Ruge WA, Chakravarti A, Langer JC: Chronic constipation due to Hirschsprung's disease and desmosis coli in a family. Pediatr Surg Int 2002;18:110–114.

167 Meier-Ruge WA: Demosis of the colon: a working hypothesis of primary chronic constipation. Eur J Pediatr Surg 1998;8:299–303.

168 Makhija PS, Magdalene KF, Babu MK: Megacystis microcolon intestinal hypoperistalsis syndrome. Indian J Pediatr 1999;66:945–949.

169 Meier-Ruge WA, Holschneider AM, Schärli AF: New pathogenetic aspects of gut dysmotility in aplastic and hypoplastic desmosis in early childhood. Pediatr Surg Int 2001;17:140–143.

170 Hübner U, Meier-Ruge W, Halsband H: Four cases of desmosis coli: severe chronic constipation, massive dilatation of the colon, and hypoperistalsis due to changes in the colonic connective-tissue net. Pediatr Surg Int 2002;18:198–203.

171 Meier-Ruge WA, Bruder E: Aplastic desmosis of the gut (aperistaltic syndrome, microcolon megacystis syndrome). Pathobiology 2005;72:42–48.

172 Meier-Ruge WA, Bruder E: The morphological characteristics of aplastic and atrophic desmosis of the intestine (in German). Pathologe 2007;28:149–154.

173 Ciftci AO, Cook RC, Van Velzen D: Megacystis microcolon intestinal hypoperistalsis syndrome: evidence of a primary myocellular defect of contractile fiber synthesis. J Pediatr Surg 1996;31:1706–1711.

174 Rolle U, O'Briain S, Pearl RH, Puri P: Megacystis-microcolon-intestinal hypoperistalsis syndrome: evidence of intestinal myopathy. Pediatr Surg Int 2002;18:2–5.

175 Piotrowsaka AP, Rolle U, Chertin B, De Caluwe D, et al: Alterations in smooth muscle contractile and cytoskeleton proteins and interstitial cells of Cajal in megacystis microcolon intestinal hypoperistalsis syndrome. J Pediatr Surg 2003;38:749–755.

176 Ruuska TH, Karikoski R, Smith VV, Milla PJ: Acquired myopathic intestinal pseudo-obstruction may be due to autoimmune enteric leiomyositis. Gastroenterology 2002;122:1133–1139.

177 Puri P, Lake BD, Gorman F, O'Donnell B, et al: Megacystis-microcolon-intestinal hypoperistalsis syndrome: a visceral myopathy. J Pediatr Surg 1983;18:64–69.

178 Moore SW, Schneider JW, Kaschula RO: Unusual variations of gasterointestinal smooth muscle abnormalities associated with chronic intestinal pseudo-obstruction. Pediatr Surg Int 2002;18:13–20.

179 Al Harbi A, Tawil K, Crankson SJ: Megacystis-microcolon-intestinal hypoperistalsis syndrome associated with megaesophagus. Pediatr Surg Int 1999;15:272–274.

180 Meier-Ruge WA, Bruder E: Atrophic desmosis of muscularis propria in the colon (hypoperistalsis syndrome). Pathobiology 2005;72:44–47.

181 Meier-Ruge WA, Bruder E: atrophic desmosis as secondary connective tissue Atrophy in muscularis propria. Pathophysiology 2005;72:78–81.

182 Meier-Ruge WA, Müller-Lobeck H, Stoss F, Bruder E: The pathogenesis of idiopathic megacolon. Eur J Gastroenterol Hepatol 2006;18:1209–1215.

183 Kapur RP, Robertson SP, Hannibal MC, Finn LS, et al: Diffuse abnormal layering of small intestinal smooth muscle is present in patients with FLNA mutations and x-linked intestinal pseudo-obstruction. Am J Surg Pathol 2010;34:1528–1543.

184 Isaacson C, Wainwright HC, Hamilton DG, OU Tim L: Hollow visceral myopathy in black South Africans. A report of 14 cases. S Afr Med J 1985;67:1015–1017.

185 Schuffler MD, Rohrmann CA, Chaffee RG, Brand DL, et al: Chronic intestinal pseudo-obstruction. A report of 27 cases and review of the literature. Medicine (Baltimore) 1981;60:173–196.

186 Martin JE, Benswon M, Swash M, Salih V, et al: Myofibroblasts in hollow visceral myopathy: the origin of gastrointestinal fibrosis. Gut 1993;34:999–1001.

187 Rode H, Brown RA, Cywes S: Degenerative hollow visceral myopathy mimicking Hirschsprung's disease; in Holschneider AM, Puri P (eds): Hirschsprung's Disease and Allied Disorders, ed 2. New York, Informa Healthcare, 2000, pp 197–210.

188 Moore SW, Schneider JW, Kaschula RD: Non-familial visceral myopathy: clinical and pathologic features of degenerative leiomyopathy. Pediatr Surg Int 2002;18:6–12.

189 Rode H, Brown RA, Numanoglu A: Degenerative hollow visceral myopathy mimicking Hirschsprung's disease; in Holschneider AM, Puri P (eds): Hirschsprung's Disease and Allied Disorders, ed 3. Berlin, Springer, 2008, pp 275–286.

190 Ducastelle T, Tranvouez JL, Lerebours E, Hemet J, et al: Hereditary visceral myopathy: an entity in idiopathic intestinal pseudo-obstruction. Gastroenterol Clin Biol 1986;10:355–363.

191 Smith VV, Milla PJ: Histological phenotypes of enteric smooth muscle disease causing functional intestinal obstruction in childhood. Histopathology 1997;31:112–122.

192 Jacobs E, Ardichvili D, Perissino A, Gottignies P, et al: A case of familial visceral myopathy with atrophy and fibrosis of the longitudinal muscle layer of the entire small bowel. Gastroenterology 1979;77:745–750.

193 Mitros FA, Schuffler MD, Teja K Anuras S: Pathologic features of familial visceral myopathy. Hum Pathol 1982;13:825–833.

194 Fitzgibbons PL, Chandrasoma PT: Familial visceral myopathy. Evidence of diffuse involvement of intestinal smooth muscles. Am J Surg Pathol 1987;11:846–854.

195 Schuffler MD, Beegle RG: Progressive systemic sclerosis of the gastrointestinal tract and hereditary hollow visceral myopathy: two distinguishable disorders of intestinal smooth muscle. Gastroenterology 179;77:664–671.

196 Wedel T, Tafazzoli K, Söllner S, Krammewr HJ, et al: Mitochondrial myopathy (complex I deficiency) associated with chronic intestinal pseudo-obstruction. Eur J Pediatr Surg 2003;13:201–205.

197 Antonucci A, Fronzoni L, Cogliandro L Cogliandro RF, et al: Chronic intestinal pseudo-obstruction. World J Gastroenterol 2008;14:2953–2961.

198 Rodrigues CA, Shepherd NA, Lennard-Jones JE, Hawley PR, et al: Familial visceral myopathy: a family with at least six involved members. Gut 1989;30:1285–1292.

199 Sipponen T, Karikoski R, Nuutinen H, Markkola A, et al: Three-generation familial visceral myopathy with alpha-actin-positive inclusion bodies in intestinal smooth muscle. J Clin Gastroenterol 2009;43:437–443.

200 Meier-Ruge WA, Bruder E: Postoperative scar stenosis of the gut. Pathobiology 2005;72:89–90.

201 Meier-Ruge WA, Bruder E: Nerve cell heterotopies in muscularis mucosae and lamina propria mucosae. Pathobiology 2005;72:64–65.

202 Meier-Ruge WA, Bruder E: The vermiform appendix and its atypical feature. Pathobiology 2005;72:66–68.

203 Karnovsky MJ, Roots L: A 'direct-coloring' thiocholine method for cholinesterase. J Histochem Cytochem 1964;12:219–221.

204 Hess R, Scarpelli DG, Pearse AGE: The cytochemical localisation of oxidative enzymes. III. Pyridine nucleotide-linked dehydrogenases. J Biophys Biochem Cytol 1958;4:753–760.

205 Nachlas MM, Tsou KC, De Souza E, Cheng CS, et al: Cytochemical demonstration of succinic dehydrogenase by use of a new p-nitrophenyl substituted ditetrazole. J Histochem Cytochem 1957;5:420–436.

206 Rolle U, Puri P: Immunohistochemical studies; in Holschneider AM, Puri P (eds): Hirschsprung's Disease and Allied Disorders. Berlin, Springer, 2008, pp 207–220.

207 Rolle U, Puri P: NADPH-diaphorase histochemistry; in Holschneider AM, Puri P (eds): Hirschsprung's Disease and Allied Disorders. Berlin, Springer, 2008, pp 199–206.

208 Tam PKH, Boyd GP: Origin, course, and ending of abnormal enteric nerve fibres in Hirschsprung disease defined by whole-mount immunohistochemistry. J Pediatr Surg 1990;25:457–461.

209 Sams VR, Bobrow LG, Happerfield L, Keeling J: Evaluation of PGP9.5 in the diagnosis of Hirschsprung's disease. J Pathol 1992;168:55–58.

210 Guinard-Samuel V, Bonnard A, De Lagausie P, Philippe-Chometta P, et al: Calretinin immunohistochemistry: a simple and efficient tool to diagnose Hirschsprung disease. Mod Pathol 2009;22:1379–1384.

211 Kapur RP, Reed RC, Finn LS, Patterson K, et al: Calretinin immunohistochemistry versus acetylcholinesterase histochemistry in the evaluation of suction rectal biopsies for Hirschsprung disease. Pediatr Dev Pathol 2009;12:6–15.

212 Noffsinger A, Fenoglio-Preiser CM, Maru D, Gilinsky N: Gastrointestinal diseases. AFIP Atlas of Nontumor Pathology, First Series Fascicle 5, 2007;783–797.

213 Faulk DL, Anuras S, Gardner GD, Mitros FA, et al: A familial visceral myopathy. Ann Intern Med 1987;89:600–606.

214 Knowles CH, Nickols CD, Feakins R, Martin JE: A systematic analysis of polyglucosan bodies in the human gastrointestinal tract in health and disease. Acta Neuropathol 2003;105:410–413.

215 Greene GM, Weldon DC, Ferrans VJ, et al: Juvenile polysaccharidosis with cardioskeletal myopathy. Arch Pathol Lab Med 1987;111:977–982.

216 Fogel S, De Tar M, Shimada H, Chandrasoma P: Sporadic visceral myopathy with inclusion bodies. A light-microscopic and ultrastructural study. Am J Surg Pathol 1993;17:473–481.

217 Di Mauro S, Schon EA: Mitochondrial respiratory-chain diseases. N Engl J Med 2003;348:2656–2668.

218 Fattoretti P, Bertoni-Freddari C, Casselli U, et al: Impaired succinic dehydrogenase activity of rat Purkinje cell mitochondria during aging. Mech Ageing Dev 1998;101:175–182.

Index

Abbreviations

AChE	acetylcholinesterase
HD	Hirschsprung's disease
HE	Hemalum-eosin
IND A	intestinal neuronal dysplasia A
IND B	intestinal neuronal dysplasia B
LDH	lactic dehydrogenase
NEC	necrotizing enterocolitis
NOS	nitroxide synthase
SDH	succinic dehydrogenase